SLEEP DISORDERS

Recent Titles in
Health and Psychology Sourcebooks

Personality Disorders: Elements, History, Examples, and Research
Vera Sonja Maass

Addictions: Elements, History, Treatments, and Research
Frances R. Frankenburg, MD, Editor

Obsessive Compulsive Disorder: Elements, History, Treatments, and Research
Leslie J. Shapiro

SLEEP DISORDERS

Elements, History, Treatments, and Research

**KATHLEEN J. SEXTON-RADEK
AND GINA GRACI**

BLOOMSBURY ACADEMIC
NEW YORK • LONDON • OXFORD • NEW DELHI • SYDNEY

BLOOMSBURY ACADEMIC

Bloomsbury Publishing Inc, 1359 Broadway, New York, NY 10018, USA
Bloomsbury Publishing Plc, 50 Bedford Square, London, WC1B 3DP, UK
Bloomsbury Publishing Ireland, 29 Earlsfort Terrace, Dublin 2, D02 AY28, Ireland

BLOOMSBURY, BLOOMSBURY ACADEMIC and the Diana logo
are trademarks of Bloomsbury Publishing Plc

First published in the United States of America 2019
Paperback edition published 2026

Copyright © Bloomsbury Publishing Inc 2026

Kathleen J. Sexton-Radek and Gina Graci have asserted their right under the Copyright, Designs and Patents Act, 1988, to be identified as Authors of this work.

Cover design: Jade Barnett
Cover image © Maria Korneeva / Getty Images

All rights reserved. No part of this publication may be: i) reproduced or transmitted in any form, electronic or mechanical, including photocopying, recording or by means of any information storage or retrieval system without prior permission in writing from the publishers; or ii) used or reproduced in any way for the training, development or operation of artificial intelligence (AI) technologies, including generative AI technologies. The rights holders expressly reserve this publication from the text and data mining exception as per Article 4(3) of the Digital Single Market Directive (EU) 2019/790.

Bloomsbury Publishing Plc does not have any control over, or responsibility for, any third-party websites referred to or in this book. All internet addresses given in this book were correct at the time of going to press. The author and publisher regret any inconvenience caused if addresses have changed or sites have ceased to exist, but can accept no responsibility for any such changes.

A catalogue record for this book is available from the British Library.

A catalog record for this book is available from the Library of Congress.

ISBN: HB: 978-1-4408-6445-2
PB: 978-1-3505-5770-3
ePDF: 978-1-4408-6446-9
eBook: 979-8-2161-4572-1

Series: Health and Psychology Sourcebooks

Typeset by Newgen KnowledgeWorks Pvt. Ltd., Chennai, India
Printed and bound in the United States of America

For product safety related questions contact productsafety@bloomsbury.com.

To find out more about our authors and books visit www.bloomsbury.com and sign up for our newsletters.

Contents

Series Foreword	vii
Introduction	ix
1 Insomnia	1
2 Sleep Apnea	23
3 Restless Legs/Periodic Limb Movement Disorder	43
4 Pain and Sleep	63
5 Parasomnias	81
6 Narcolepsy	95
7 Pediatric Sleep	109
8 Student Sleep	123
9 Oncology and Sleep	131
10 Dreaming as a Psychological Process	149
Further Resources	163
Index	165

Series Foreword

An understanding of both physical diseases and mental disorders is vital to each of us, as sickness of body and mind touches every one of us throughout our lives personally; with family, friends, and associates; and in our immediate and greater society. Yet the cacophony of existing information sources—from piecemeal and poorly sourced websites to dense academic tomes—can make acquiring accurate, accessible, and objective facts a complicated venture. This series is a solution to that dilemma.

The *Health and Psychology Sourcebooks* series addresses physical, psychological, and environmental conditions that threaten human health and well-being. These books are designed to accessibly and reliably fulfill the needs of students and researchers at community and undergraduate college levels, whether one is seeking vetted information needed for core or elective courses, papers and publications, or personal enlightenment.

Each volume presents a topic in health or psychology and explains the symptoms, diagnosis, incidence, development, causes, treatments, and related theory. Vignettes illustrate how the disease or disorder and its associated difficulties present in varied people and scenarios. History and classic as well as emerging research are detailed. Where controversy is present, that is discussed. Each volume also offers resources for further reading.

Introduction

We spend so much of our human lives sleeping, but we have not mastered how to sleep "smart." While we have smart telephones, televisions, and other devices, we lack in our ability to develop smart sleep behaviors. We have wrist watches that monitor heart rate and steps taken during the day and number of hours slept with number of awakenings. These devices tell us how much of our sleep occurs in the different stages of sleep. While these devices are focused on staying healthy and fit, we need to ensure that we are prioritizing healthy sleep habits and allocating enough time for sleep.

Sleep is a phenomenon common to all human beings, and approximately one-third of our lives is spent asleep. Yet there are so many things that can influence sleep, such as behaviors, illness or disease, medications, amount of light exposure, environmental exposures, and/or traveling across time zones. Things we do during the day or evening can also influence our sleep. For instance, for some individuals, getting into bed and surfing the internet can be a mentally stimulating activity that is not conducive to sleep. Individuals are encouraged to learn about and implement healthy sleep behaviors so that they do not experience sleep disturbance or sleep loss.

Sleep is critical for the brain and the body. The proper amount of sleep helps with improved thinking, better focus, and faster reflexes. It also interacts with how the body functions, immune function, and hormonal interaction with cellular repair and overall energy use. Sleep varies by age and other factors, but the average amount of adult sleep is seven to eight hours per night. Quantity of sleep is important, but quality of sleep is also important.

Our book addresses sleep disorders and methods for improving sleep. In 2015, the Joint Consensus Statement of the American Academy of Sleep Medicine and Sleep Research Society recommended the amount of sleep for healthy adults (Watson et al., 2015). The results of the panel demonstrated that seven to nine hours sleep, by consensus, is necessary for good health. Sleep deprivation can have dire consequences to health, performance, and safety.

What is a sleep disorder? Sleep disorders are defined when the individual's sleep pattern is aberrant to a typical pattern. The causes are varied and can include biological, behavioral, and environmental factors. Insomnia is the most reported sleep disorder and is defined as difficulty initiating and maintaining sleep. The most common sleep disorder diagnosed in a sleep laboratory or facility is obstructive sleep apnea. It is defined as a sleep-related breathing disorder that involves a decrease or complete halt in airflow despite an ongoing effort to breathe (American Academy of Sleep Medicine [AASM], 2020).

In our book, we have selected common sleep disorders with explanations in each chapter. We've also included a society and individual perspective so that the reader can better understand the impact of the sleep disorder on an individual's sleep.

References

American Academy of Sleep Medicine. 2020. *Sleep apnea—Overview and facts*. http://sleepeducation.org/essentials-in-sleep/sleep-apnea.

N. F. Watson, M. S. Badr, G. Belenky, D. L. Bliwise, O. M. Buxton, D. Buysse, et al. (2015). Joint consensus statement of the American Academy of Sleep Medicine and Sleep Research Society on the recommended amount of sleep for a healthy adult: Methodology and discussion. *Sleep, 38*(8), 1161–1183. https://doi.org/doi: 10.5665/sleep.4886

CHAPTER 1

Insomnia

Sleep is a phenomenon common to all human beings, and approximately one-third of our lives is spent asleep. Sleep has been defined as an altered state of consciousness with reduced responsiveness to external stimuli (Graci & Sexton-Radek, 2005; Hodgson, 1991; Wilson-Barnett, Batehup, & Fordam, 1988, 148–81). The true purpose of sleep remains unknown, but hypotheses abound (Benington, 2000). Sleep has been postulated to facilitate learning and memory consolidation (Blissitt, 2001; Sejnowski & Destexhe, 2000), maintenance of synaptic efficacy (Krueger & Obal, 1993), immunologic restoration (Born, Lange, Hansen, Molle, & Fehm, 1997), and overall homeostasis (Benington, 2000). Yet recent reviews have found inconclusive results for these claims (Maquet, 2001; Siegel, 2001). Nevertheless, it appears that sleep serves an important restorative function and is composed of many complex behavioral and physiological processes (Graci & Sexton-Radek, 2005).

Review of Sleep Stages

Sleep architecture refers to the various stages in the sleep-wake cycle, typically defined by electroencephalogram (EEG) recording. Graci and Sexton-Radek (2005) summarized rapid eye movement (REM) and non-REM (NREM) sleep stages. In healthy individuals without sleep problems, these stages occur in a regular pattern throughout a 24-hour period. There are two types of sleep: dream/REM and NREM sleep. The first, dream or REM sleep, occurs every 1.5 hours throughout the sleep interval, or 18–25% of the sleep period. REM periods vary in length from several minutes to more than an hour. REM sleep has a characteristic physiological pattern distinguished by the lateral saccadic rhythm of the eyes, absence of muscle movement, and heightened cardiovascular arousal. Studies of self-reported REM periods have revealed the changing themes of dreams from everyday events to surreal wish fantasies toward the end of the sleep period.

In contrast, NREM sleep occupies a greater portion of the sleep period. NREM is further subdivided into stages 1, 2, 3, and 4 with corresponding physiological activity to each. Stage 1 is considered light sleep and is estimated to make up some 5% of the sleep period. Stage 2 sleep is about 60% of the sleep intervals and is formally considered "sleep." Stages 3 and 4 are often collapsed together and are classified as deep sleep, a physiological event characterized by slow brain wave patterns and increased immune system activity. Deep sleep makes up approximately 10–15% of the sleep period.

A night of sleep is characterized as a predicted pattern of sleep onset followed by stage 1 sleep onset, and then a progression to stages 2, 3, and 4. On or slightly before 90 minutes after sleep onset, the first REM episode occurs (four to five REM episodes occur per night). Following this, the cycle repeats itself in this progression with four cycles of sleep per night. An excess or deficit in the amount of a type of sleep, a misordering of the timing of sleep, or an intrusion of sleep represents conditions for further study to determine sleep disorder.

Insomnia

It is estimated that 35% of the general population complain of sleep disturbances that meet insomnia criteria. The *International Classification System of Sleep Disorders (ICSD)* (Sateia, 2014) and the *Diagnostic and Statistical Manual of Mental Disorders*, Fifth Edition (*DSM-5*) are the two classification systems currently used for diagnosing insomnia. Insomnia is defined in the *DSM-5* as difficulty initiating or maintaining sleep or nonrestorative sleep with sleep disruption occurring at least three times per week for a period of at least three months. This type of sleep disruption causes clinically significant distress or impairment in social, occupational, or other important areas of functioning (American Psychiatric Association [APA], 2013). The most prominent feature of insomnia remains the complaint of poor sleep, either in inadequate duration or in quality, which impacts quality of life, mood, energy, and daytime functioning (Graci & Sexton-Radek, 2005; Morin, 2000). The disruption can be a delay in falling asleep (sleep initiation), an inability to maintain sleep throughout the night, and early morning waking with difficulty returning to sleep. These types of sleep disruption in either quality or quantity of sleep can cause physical and emotional impairment, especially if the disruption becomes chronic. In both laboratory and natural settings, sleep deprivation following insomnia has been associated with a decline in cognitive function, inability to engage in work or recreational activities, loss of hedonic capacity, and a sharp decline in quality of life, as well as alterations to immune and neuroendocrine function (Ehrenberg, 2000; Lamberg, 2000; Savard et al., 1999).

Chronic insomnia needs to be appropriately diagnosed and addressed by clinicians because it is a major risk factor for major depression (Kryger, Roth, & Dement, 2001; Sateia, Doghramji, Hauri, & Morin, 2000) and also influences other morbidities (Graci & Sexton-Radek, 2005). Clinicians must consider a detailed history of the nature, duration, severity, and course of the insomnia complaint and investigate the contribution of psychological, medical, behavioral, and environmental factors (Graci & Sexton-Radek, 2005; Mills & Graci, 2004; Morin, 2000).

Several risk factors for insomnia need to be addressed. Insomnia is more common among females, older individuals, and the depressed or anxious (Aldrich, 2000; Morin & Ware, 1996; National Sleep Foundation, 2017; Savard, Simard, Blanchet, Ivers, & Morin, 2001). Additionally, low socioeconomic status, chronic medical illness, pain syndromes, low education, recent life stressors, certain medications, and alcohol use are associated with insomnia complaints.

Morin (1993, 2004) is a complete resource of the conceptualization, assessment, and treatment of insomnia. Once a pattern of sleep disturbance has been set, several factors serve to maintain that disturbance. Of course, the continuing use of maladaptive sleep behaviors, napping during the daytime, spending excessive amount of time in bed, and maintaining an irregular sleep-wake cycle, will both maintain and possibly worsen sleep disturbances (Morin, 1993). If chronic exposure to environmental factors occurs, sleep disturbance will most likely occur. Environmental factors include but are not limited to noise, light, temperature (too hot/too cold), and/or uncomfortable beds.

Other major factors in the continuance of sleep problems are patients' faulty beliefs and attitudes about sleep and sleep disturbance (Savard & Morin, 2001). For instance, some patients believe that eight hours of continuous sleep each night is necessary to maintain daily functioning and maintain health. However, there is wide variability in nightly sleep patterns. If patients can sleep as much or as often as necessary or desired, the normal range of sleep time among healthy individuals ranges from six hours to ten hours or more (Lee, 1997). Further, there appears to be no evidence that occasional loss of sleep has any lasting effect, and yet, to an insomniac, loss of sleep or perceived loss of sleep can have debilitating psychological effects. Sleep disturbance often elicits anxiety about continued sleep disturbance, leaving patients lying in bed, worrying about whether they will get to sleep or get enough sleep in the coming night. Such worry and anxiety further contribute to sleep disturbances (Graci & Sexton-Radek, 2005). Reduction of the sustained arousal that is characteristic of insomnia must be the focus of treatment (Spielman & Anderson, 1999).

Treatment approaches for insomnia have been individual therapy, group therapy, and therapeutic-like education (e.g., sleep hygiene, stimulus control therapies), cognitive behavioral therapy, and medication management. The focus of these treatment approaches has been in terms of providing education about insomnia, maintaining sleep schedules, or seeking support care or medical/therapeutic care.

Long-Term Effects of Insomnia

Insomnia has many causes, and the effects of insomnia can impair many areas of life. The behaviors (i.e., poor sleep hygiene) that can lead to insomnia can negatively impact one's overall functioning. Individuals who complain of insomnia often fear losing their jobs or report having poor work performance due to sleepiness and difficulties with concentration. Daytime sleepiness can lead to job-related injuries, automobile accidents, and a decrease in quality of life.

Therapeutic Approaches for Insomnia Management

It is widely agreed that effective treatment of insomnia must assume a multidisciplinary approach in which physiological, psychological, behavioral, and environmental interventions receive equal emphasis. Approximately 70–80% of patients treated with nonpharmacological interventions benefit from treatment (Morin, 1999b, 2003, 2004; Morin & Azrin, 1987, 1988; Morin, Bastien, & Savard, 2003). For patients with chronic primary insomnia, nonpharmacological treatments are likely to reduce sleep onset and/or wake after sleep onset to less than 30 minutes, with sleep quality and satisfaction scores significantly increasing (Morin, 1999a, 1999b). Three treatments meet the APA criteria for empirically supported behavioral treatments for insomnia: stimulus control therapy, progressive muscle relaxation, and paradoxical intention.

Three other treatments meet APA criteria for probably efficacious treatments: sleep restriction, biofeedback, and multifaceted cognitive behavioral therapy. Cognitive behavioral therapy (CBT) has been found to show much more long-lasting improvements following treatment than pharmacological agents in treating chronic primary insomnias (Edinger, Wohlgemuth, Radtke, Marsh, & Quillian, 2001) because CBT is able to target the underlying problem, whereas termination of pharmacological agents can cause a rebound of the initial sleep difficulties (Graci & Sexton-Radek, 2005).

Insomnia Treatment Approaches

Cognitive Treatment Approaches

Cognitive Behavioral Therapy. In addition to these three specific behavioral strategies, a more general cognitive behavioral approach is implemented for insomnia treatment (Graci & Sexton-Radek, 2005). For example, many patients who have difficulty sleeping begin to worry about their lack of sleep and the nightly struggle to achieve a restful sleep, which increases anxiety.

- Patients may ruminate more about their sleep patterns than the current psychosocial stressors they are experiencing.
- They begin to develop cognitions that only amplify the problem.
- Sleep difficulties may be seen as potential contributors to ongoing problems.

As a result, patients become more concerned about the loss of sleep and its potential impact on health, financial security, job performance, and so on. For instance, a patient presented with complaints of difficulty falling sleep at night and awakening early in the morning without the ability to return to sleep. She would ruminate at night about not being able to fall asleep and how this lack of sleep would negatively impact her job performance and result in termination. How would she be able to support her family or be able to afford college for her children with the loss of income? The focus of treatment is challenging the veracity of these "beliefs" and encouraging alternative thoughts. Once alternative thoughts are identified, the patient can then compare the "faulty beliefs" to the alternative thoughts.

Morin (1993) advises the use of this three-step process: first, identify patient-specific dysfunctional cognitions; second, confront and challenge their validity; and third, replace them with more adaptive and rational substitutes. These steps help alleviate excessive worry about sleep and, in turn, reduce daytime worries that are accumulated and lead to heightened cognitive activity (i.e., worry).

Behavioral Treatment Approaches

Any behavioral treatment strategy for insomnia needs to begin with patient education. The primary focus is to teach patients how to recognize sleep problems and their contributions to those sleep problems (e.g., drinking caffeine before bedtime) so that they can help restore their sleep with the help of their provider teams. Education is the key to assisting patients to replace disruptive sleep behaviors with healthy sleep behaviors.

The three general behavioral approaches to insomnia treatment focus on sleep hygiene (Hauri, 1993, 2000), stimulus control, and sleep restriction therapies (Graci & Sexton-Radek, 2005; Manber & Kuo, 2002). After a brief educational session with a trained sleep specialist who teaches the patient appropriate (adaptive) sleep behaviors, the patent initiates these behaviors at home. During subsequent clinic visits, a follow-up inquiry is made as to how successful implementation of the behaviors has been, and specific barriers to achieving the goals of treatment are explored. All three treatment approaches require that patients observe their sleep patterns as they instigate these changes while monitoring their sleep/rest/wake times using a sleep self-monitoring form (i.e., sleep diary) or other assessment instrument. Graci and Sexton-Radek (2005) and Sexton-Radek and Graci (2009) illustrate key sleep behavior treatment regimens.

Sleep Hygiene. Sleep hygiene refers to the organization of activities to minimize sleep disturbance. Typically, it incorporates the following behaviors:

- Reduce the intake of nicotine, caffeine, and other stimulants.
- If stimulants must be taken, avoid them in the afternoon or evening.
- Avoid alcohol near bedtime.
- Keep a regular daytime schedule for work, rest, meals, treatment, exercise, and other daily activities.
- Do strenuous exercises only in the earlier part of the day rather than in the late afternoon or evening.

Stimulus Control. The overall goal of stimulus control is to train the patients, through a learning paradigm, to associate the bed with sleeping and sleeping with the bed. In addition, patients learn to "set" their sleep-wake cycle. To achieve these goals, the following behaviors are suggested:

- Go to bed only when sleepy.
- Do not engage in activity in bed other than sleep (sexual activity is an exception); in other words, reading, eating, watching television, or completing homework is not to be done in bed but in another area of the home.
- If sleep does not come within 15 or 20 minutes of retiring at night, get out of bed and engage in relaxing behavior, returning to bed only when sleepy (this may be repeated as often as needed throughout the night).
- Wake at the same time every day, regardless of the amount of sleep achieved during the night.
- Avoid daytime naps.

Sleep Restriction. The patient maintains a sleep log to establish baseline sleep times following the onset of sleep disturbance to determine sleep efficiency. In other words, if the patient spends eight hours in bed, but only achieves four hours of sleep, on average, the sleep efficiency is four out of eight, or 50%. The patient is then directed to spend only four hours in bed each night until a sleep efficiency of 90% or more (3.6 hours) is achieved. Then a half hour is added to the allotted time in bed, and this sleep schedule is maintained until the patient again achieves a sleep efficiency of 90%. This pattern is followed until the patient reaches the target sleep time.

In addition to cognitive behavioral therapy, patients may also benefit from understanding and utilizing a variety of relaxation techniques. These techniques may range from relatively simple techniques that require three to five minutes of teaching to much more complex shifts in the patients' views of life, which can consume two months or more of teaching. Graci and Sexton-Radek (2005) summarize some of these techniques:

- Progressive muscle relaxation. In this technique, patients learn to stretch and relax successive areas of the body in an effort to "teach" the body what relaxation feels like. For example, a patient is told to squint his or her eyes as tightly as possible, keeping them closed for a count of five, and then relaxing them completely. This is repeated two or three times, and then the patient moves to another area of close proximity, such as the mouth. He or she stretches the mouth open as

tightly as possible for a count of five, and then releases the muscles, allowing the mouth muscles to relax. The patient repeats this two or three times, and then moves on to the neck, repeating this procedure in other bodily areas, all the way down to the toes.
- Biofeedback. Biofeedback allows the patient to control body temperature and tension using an electronic feedback system. This technique requires both equipment and training and is not likely to benefit patients who have multiple medical problems to address. A biofeedback professional is required to teach this.
- Guided imagery. This technique focuses on directing a patient to sit or lie comfortably and take two or three deep breaths with eyes closed. A certified guided imagery therapist needs to train the patient. The technique starts by asking the patient to choose a "safe" image or memory, or the professional may suggest a peaceful scene. While the professional describes the peaceful scene, a patient is "dropped into" the scene with progressively broader awareness. In summary, the patient uses visual, auditory, olfactory, and tactual senses (e.g., if at the beach, the visual scenery of ocean, waves, and sand, as well as the sound of crashing waves, the sound of birds, the smell of the salt of the ocean, and the feel of the sand between the fingers). Finally, the patient is asked to imagine what it feels like to be in the scene. He or she is encouraged to feel peaceful, relaxed, calm, satisfied, and without pain. After the certified therapist leads the patient through this process once or twice, a tape of one of the sessions can be provided for the patient to use at home before retiring for the evening.

Hypnosis in the Treatment of Insomnia

Clinical hypnosis is a safe and effective method of treating insomnia because it allows the clinician to gain access to the underlying problem (Modlin, 2002). Self-hypnosis is considered a voluntary relaxation technique (Dement & Vaughan, 2000) that is like meditation in that it can ease the body and mind into preparing for sleep (Kryger 2004). Hypnosis and self-hypnosis offer rapid methods for managing anxiety and worry, facilitating deep relaxation, controlling mental overactivity and decreasing physiological arousal, which are cardinal symptoms of insomnia (Bauer & McCanne, 1980; Hammond, 1990).

There are somatically based insomnias but these have been found to be unamenable to hypnotic interventions (Weitzenhoffer, 2000). Some of the psychological insomnias (i.e., either individuals become upset prior to sleep onset, or they wake up and experience difficulty returning to sleep because they become anxious about not sleeping or losing sleep) are very amenable to hypnotism.

Hypnotic scripts are illustrated in the following examples. The reader is cautioned that before hypnotic scripts may be utilized, sleep hygiene, stimulus control therapy, sleep restriction, and cognitive therapy techniques need to be taught to the patient. Once one or all these techniques are taught to the patient, induction techniques, followed by deepening techniques are implemented, and then the hypnotic suggestions, which are designed to focus on improving quality and duration of sleep. The hypnotic suggestions can include sleep hygiene, stimulus control, sleep restriction, and cognitive therapy techniques. The last step is to apply awakening techniques (Graci & Hardie, 2007).

Both examples may be used after induction or deepening suggestions have been implemented, or you may use either of these examples as a deepening technique. You may add on additional hypnotic suggestions or apply awakening suggestions for returning to alertness.

Example 1

Ensure that the patient has engaged in calming presleep activities prior to retiring for bed. Make sure that the bedroom is free of tension and worry.

Before you retire for bed, you will make sure that your bedroom is free of tension and worry. Allow yourself to begin to feel relaxation and prepare your body for slumber by freeing yourself from any anxiety or distraction from television, mobile phone, or computer and allow yourself to focus your attention on calming the body down. Begin to turn off lights, remove any distractions, and quiet your mind. As you get into bed, you will automatically begin to unwind and relax. You will notice changes in your breathing as it becomes deeper and more relaxed. You are aware of how intuitively you begin to fall asleep. Be confident that your body knows how to fall asleep and stay asleep and rest. You will be surprised at how well you are able to fall deeply asleep. You will be able to maintain sleep through the night and will feel refreshed and rested. When you wake up, your body will recognize the good feeling of restful sleep and the benefits from consolidated, deep sleep. You will notice how easily you adapt to healthy undisturbed sleep. You feel confident in knowing that as you sleep, your body is building strength and immunity. You can know how profoundly your body benefits from deep, deep, relaxing sleep and the feeling of waking up feeling refreshed and rested.

Example 2

I want you to visualize that your bedroom is a place of safety that does not include distractions or worry. Imagine walking toward your bedroom. You give yourself permission to leave all concerns or anything that is troubling you outside of your bedroom. When you awaken in the morning, you can retrieve these worries or troubles when you leave your bedroom. There is no need to bring these thoughts into your bedroom because bedroom is a safe haven. It is your personal safety zone. It is here that you can experience peace, calm, comfort, and safety.

You see that your bedroom door is getting closer and closer, and you notice that you are feeling calmer and more relaxed. You have nothing concerning on your mind as you approach your bedroom, and this feeling of profound relaxation becomes deeper and deeper, especially as you walk into your bedroom. You notice that you are feeling more relaxed, more secure, and calmer as you approach your bed. Your limbs are growing heavier and heavier as you lie on your bed and feel the covers of your bed. As you get into bed, you notice how comfortable and calm you feel lying in your bed. Your mind is profoundly quiet, and you feel safe and relaxed. Your eyelids are beginning to get heavier and heavier, and you welcome this heaviness.

When you are ready, your eyelids close. You notice that you are free of any emotional or physical discomfort and feel comfortable. You don't have any worries or concerns, because your mind is very quiet and calm. You are feeling so sleepy that you can no longer keep your eyelids open, and you welcome this feeling of profound sleep. There is no need to check the clock because your body knows how to fall asleep, how to maintain sleep, and how to wake up when the body is ready to wake up. It is important to remember that when your body is ready to sleep, it will sleep. You continue to welcome this experience of deep and profound sleep. If you awaken during the night, you will easily return to sleep even if you have gotten up to use the bathroom, because your body knows how to sleep. You feel calm, peaceful, safe, and very, very sleepy. You know that your body knows how to sleep because you have done it since you were a child. It is automatic; much like a child, you welcome sleep, and your body will wake when it has had enough sleep. Keep your bedtimes and waketime, even on the weekends at the same time . . . You can master deep, profound, restorative sleep, just as you have the ability to manage the day-to-day activities of your life right now. When you awake in the morning, you will feel refreshed, peaceful, full of energy and ready to start your day.

Case Studies

The following case scenarios illustrate different situations in which patients presented with sleep issues related to illness and poor sleep hygiene. Most of the time, change in the patients' behavior must occur to address and treat the sleep disorders/complaints. Generally, the change involves (but is not limited to) scheduling consistent bed and wake times, engaging in proper sleep hygiene behaviors, challenging faulty beliefs about sleep (e.g., I will die if I do not get a good night's sleep), and restricting sleep times to improve sleep quality and duration of sleep.

Case Study: Patient with Life-Threatening Illness

Ollie is a 55-year-old athletic (runner and cyclist) male who was diagnosed with human immunodeficiency virus (HIV) in 2010. Ollie had been asymptomatic; however, a recent follow-up appointment showed that his current HIV medication was not working, and his T-cell count was decreasing. He also had significant muscle wasting in his legs, which was a side effect of his HIV medications.

He was referred by his infectious disease physician because Ollie was complaining of difficulty falling asleep and staying asleep. During his first sleep appointment, the clinician reviewed Ollie's daily routine as well as his eating and exercising behaviors. Ollie stated that he was a mortgage broker, business had not been doing well, and he was afraid he would lose his job and health insurance. When asked to rate his level of worry about losing his job, he rated it at 10/10, meaning that his level of worry was the highest on a rating scale of 1–10.

Additionally, when his daily routine was explored, Ollie explained that he would wake up at 6:00 a.m. and have three to four cups of coffee prior to arriving at his job at about 9:00 a.m. He also drank two to four cups of coffee between the hours of 1:00 p.m. and 3:00 p.m. When he arrived at home, he watched television and fell asleep while watching a television show. On average, he slept between 30 and 90 minutes.

He also stated that he has been in a relationship that has been argumentative, and his partner often got drunk and violent. While Ollie states that he loves his partner, he is contemplating breaking up because he recognizes that the relationship is not healthy. He admits to being fearful that no one will want to be with him because of his HIV status, so he tends to "put up with" his partners dysfunctional behaviors.

He prepares to go to bed at around 9:30 p.m. and lies in bed, thinking about his work, health, and relationship. He tosses and turns for about

2 hours and consistently worries that he needs to sleep or he will not feel well during the day, and being sleepy could impact his work performance. He also worries that not sleeping will further impair his immune system.

His first appointment lasted approximately 1.5 hours, and at the end of the session, Ollie was given a sleep diary to record his habits, including, but not limited to, the time he gets into bed, sleep onset time, his emotions, sleep behaviors, number of times awakening, and total sleep time, as well as whether he wakes up feeling refreshed. Ollie stated that he was willing to try anything but did not have a lot of faith in being able to restore his sleep. He stated that he would complete the sleep diary every day and that it would remain with him throughout the day so that he could document stressful events that occurred during the day, as well as the time he took his medications, and so on. It is important to note that none of Ollie's current medications affect timing of sleep (when to fall asleep) and sleep duration (length of sleep).

Ollie returned for his second appointment one week later, and he seemed more anxious and frustrated than during his initial visit. He stated that he completed the sleep diary daily, but the diary made him more aware of how much he was not sleeping, and this new awareness made him anxious throughout the day and night. He stated that he was constantly thinking about not sleeping and how much he was hurting his immune system. When asked, "What are you doing to relax yourself?" he stated that he has been drinking a "couple of beers" before bedtime.

Upon review of his sleep diary, Ollie was engaging in behaviors that were not conducive to sleep. For instance, he was drinking caffeine after 12:00 p.m., working out two hours before bedtime, drinking alcohol one to two hours before bedtime, ruminating on not been able to sleep and how his lack of sleep is negatively impacting his health, and napping in the evening hours, all of which can contribute to delaying sleep onset and maintaining sleep. Ollie was clearly engaging in poor sleep hygiene behaviors; he had to learn about not only eliminating stimulating activities but also ingesting stimulating substances such as caffeine and alcohol. Education was the key focus in trying to restore healthy sleep behaviors. Ollie was somewhat reluctant to eliminate caffeine after noon, not drink alcohol six to eight hours before bedtime, and exercise in the morning prior to going to work.

Review of his sleep diary suggested that Ollie's bedtime is around 11:00 p.m. and that getting into bed at nine o'clock will lead to tossing and turning and increasing his anxiety about not being able to fall asleep. Treatment focused on a combined CBT, sleep hygiene, sleep restriction, and stimulus control therapies. Ollie needed to engage in calming and relaxing behaviors one hour before bedtime. If he was not feeling sleepy at eleven, he was not to go to bed but remain in another room and continue to engage in relaxing, calming behaviors. If watching television or reading a book is mentally stimulating, patients are advised to not engage in these behaviors. Texting or going on the internet is a mentally stimulating activity that is to be avoided for those who have difficulty initiating and staying asleep. Last, relationship counseling and individual therapy were recommended, and Ollie agreed to find and participate in both types of therapy.

At appointment three, Ollie revealed that he found both an individual and relationship psychologist. He was having a hard time giving up caffeine, alcohol, and napping. He stated that he was staying in bed even when he felt alert and remained in bed even though he couldn't sleep. Sleep restriction therapy was implemented to address staying in bed when he is not sleepy.

By appointment four, progress was being made with eliminating caffeine, alcohol, and napping. However, Ollie found that he was very sleepy during the day. He was listening to music until he felt sleepy and returned to bed. If he didn't fall asleep and felt he could not sleep, he returned to his living room and listened to music until he felt sleepy and went back to bed. His sleep diary revealed that over the course of one week, he was able to shorten his time to sleep onset (he was falling asleep closer to 11:00 p.m.) and staying asleep, aside from normal nighttime bathroom awakenings. He was also able to return to sleep easier than he had been.

At appointment five, Ollie revealed that individual therapy was very beneficial to him because he was addressing his fears regarding his health, employment, and self-worth. He stated that therapy was a lot of work because he had to look at himself and at the parts of himself that he did not like. He also stated that the relationship therapy was not effective because his partner did not show up for the last two sessions. Ollie's sleep diary showed that he had disruptive sleep for three days after he attended an office party and consumed two or three beers over the course of the evening. He was unable to fall asleep and fell back to his "old" behaviors of worrying that his lack of sleep was affecting is health, and so on. It took him three nights to get his sleep back on track.

At appointment six, Ollie's sleep diary revealed that he was sleeping six to seven hours, on average, per night and was waking up feeling more refreshed. He stated that exercising when he woke up has been helpful because he feels more energetic during the day; when he starts to feel sleepy at work, he gets up and walks outside for a breath of fresh air. While he continued to find it difficult to avoid napping, his sleep diary revealed that he was going to bed between 10:15 and 10:30 and achieving 7.5 hours of sleep. He has also seen a nutritionist to ensure that he is eating healthy foods to help his immune functioning. He stated that the combination of therapies, nutrition, and sleep therapy has been very helpful in helping him worry less and focus on the present. His company is downsizing, but his job is secure for now. He also stated that his infectious disease doctor suggested that he speak with a social worker regarding his employment concerns and the potential loss of health insurance. He stated that meeting with the social worker was also beneficial and removed some of the employment stress.

At appointment seven, review of Ollie's sleep diary revealed that he continued to sleep 6–7.5 hours a night and was eating healthier since he started working with his nutritionist. He cut down on sugar and caffeine intake and continued to feel good. Ollie stated that he felt he had the sleep skills to keep his sleep on schedule and that, if there is an issue, he knows how to get back on track. If he was unsuccessful, he would schedule a follow-up visit.

At appointment eight, six months later, Ollie stated that his health remained stable and that he had some difficulty with falling and staying asleep, primarily because he broke up with his partner. Initially, it was very difficult because he felt unlovable, but he was able to work through some of these low feelings of self-worth and realize that he would rather be alone than in a relationship that is violent and full of turmoil. The appointment focused on reviewing his six months of sleep diaries (he continued to complete them) and to provide sleep education in situations where his sleep schedule was thrown off.

Overall, Ollie was able to achieve waking up with refreshed sleep, keeping consistent bed and wake times, and adhering to sleep hygiene principles for healthy sleeping. It took approximately one year with a combination of working with a sleep clinician and a psychologist to achieve progress with getting Ollie to achieve a good night sleep. Ollie stated that he accepted his HIV status and his outlook changed from being "dark and negative" about his future to being happy to participate in life on a daily basis.

Case Study: Nocturnal Texting
Cindy is a 33-year-old graphic designer who presented to the sleep clinic with difficulties falling asleep. Aside from a diagnosis of endometriosis, her medical history is benign. She is a long-distance runner (running

eight miles daily), participates in yoga, and is on a city community softball league. She stated that she broke up with her last boyfriend six months prior and had not been dating anyone. She is close to her siblings, two younger sisters and an older brother. Her parents live close by, and she visits them once a week. She has no financial concerns and does not describe herself as an anxious person. She stated that she feels lonely occasionally because many of her friends are in relationships, and she often turns down social events because she does not want to be "the third wheel."

Cindy stated that she goes to bed between 11:00 p.m. and 12:00 a.m. but does not fall asleep until 2:00 a.m., and she wakes up at 7:00 a.m. (sleep duration of approximately five hours). She stated that she does not wake up feeling refreshed and is often tired during the day. She lives close to her work, so she is able to sleep later before she has to arrive at work at 8:00 a.m. Cindy was given a sleep diary to complete, and an appointment was scheduled for one week later.

At her second appointment, Cindy's sleep diary was reviewed and revealed that she does not drink caffeine after ten o'clock in the morning and exercises at the gym during her lunch hour. She eats dinner between 5:00 and 6:00 p.m. daily. The sleep diary revealed no alcohol intake. Cindy watches television from 7:00 to 10:00 p.m., and then starts texting and spending time on social websites until she can fall asleep.

Cindy's sleep disturbance is related to her texting and going on social websites, both of which are mentally stimulating activities. Cindy was asked what types of activities she found calming and relaxing, and she stated reading a book, praying, or listening to music. For Cindy, reading a book was not a mentally stimulating activity. She was advised to not to text or go on the internet for at least two hours before bedtime. She stated that giving up both activities would be difficult.

At appointment three, Cindy's sleep diary revealed that she did not refrain from texting or using the internet for two hours before bedtime. When queried about her avoidance, she stated that she was used to engaging in these activities to help clear her head. Despite explaining that texting, and so on, are mentally stimulating, she appeared reluctant to change her behaviors but stated that she would try.

Three days after Cindy's third appointment, she called the clinic stating that she was unsuccessful in giving up her texting/internet because she became anxious. When asked what she was doing instead, she stated nothing—she was just focusing on not wanting to text/use the internet. Cindy was encouraged to either pray, read, or listen to music, and she said that she would try.

At appointment four, Cindy reported falling asleep in her living room while listening to music. Cindy was advised to go to her bedroom as soon as she feels sleepy; she agreed. Despite the three days that Cindy reported texting or using the internet, the remainder of the days showed a slight improvement in sleep.

At appointment five, her sleep diary revealed that she continued to fall asleep while listening to music. She stated that sleep just "happens," and she did not even realize that she was falling asleep. Review of her sleep diary suggested that Cindy's bedtime needed to be changed from 11:00 p.m. to 10:30 p.m. She agreed to make this switch and was told to just go to her bed and try to fall asleep if she felt sleepy prior to 10:30. If she was unable to fall asleep within 5–10 minutes, she was to return to the living room until she felt sleepy and then return to bed.

At appointment six, Cindy stated that she believed her sleep schedule was working. She stated that on four of seven nights, she was able to fall asleep at around 10:30 p.m. in her bed. She stated that on three nights, she fell asleep on the couch at around ten o'clock. She was advised to try to move her bedtime to 10:00 p.m. She agreed.

At appointment seven, her sleep diary revealed that Cindy was sleeping, on average, 8.5–9 hours a night and was feeling good. She reported feeling refreshed upon awakening and denied feeling sleepy during the day. She also stated that she was given a promotion and was very happy with her job.

In summary, by having Cindy eliminate the texting and surfing the internet prior to bedtime, she was able to engage in healthy, sleep-promoting behaviors that allowed her to achieve a good night's sleep and wake up feeling energized. While Cindy initially struggled with giving up the nighttime texting, she was able to move the texting to the time before and during dinner. She was told to stop texting and surfing the internet by 7:00–8:00 p.m., which was not a problem for her once she got used to the change. She was not denied texting; rather, she changed the hours of texting. She reported that it felt "good to have a clear head and relaxing body." She stated that she had not felt "this level of calm" in her life before. She stopped using her sleep diary once she was able to repeatedly achieve restful sleep.

Case Study: Poor Sleep Hygiene
Susie was a mother of three children under the age of ten and reported feeling anxious at night and being unable to sleep. She was unable to describe what was causing the anxiety or any thoughts or associations that would provoke the anxiety. She has to drive her children to school

in the morning and pick them up after school. In between those times, Susie reported napping during the day. She stated that she often missed out on having lunch with her friends because she was too sleepy. She noticed that there was a trend in missing out on social activities and even some events with her husband and children. Susie denied experiencing depression and was unwilling to change her sleep behaviors.

Susie was referred to the sleep clinic by her general practitioner to find the cause of her excessive daytime sleepiness. Results of the intake suggested that Susie's sleepiness was related to being sleep deprived, caused by hyperarousal at night. She denied symptoms related to another sleep disorder, and her bed partner was interviewed to determine if she had pauses in her breathing during the night (e.g., obstructive sleep apnea), snoring with arousals, leg movements, and so on. The interview was negative for a diagnosis of another type of sleep disorder. Susan refused to complete a sleep diary and did not want to attend "sleep sessions."

A week after her intake, her general physician called and asked if she would benefit from hypnosis. Based on complaints of nocturnal hyperarousal and a lack of other symptoms of a sleep disorder, Susie was referred to a sleep doctor who is trained in hypnosis. No further follow-up was provided by her physician.

For patients who do not have additional sleep disorders other than experiencing the nocturnal hyperarousal associated with insomnia, hypnosis may be effective in those patients who are suggestive to hypnosis.

Those insomniacs who turn to sleep medications (over the counter or prescription) are often not addressing the real cause of the sleep problem. These "medications" are a quick fix, and many individuals report having problems with sleep if they skip a night of taking their "medication."

Case Study: Living with a Parent Who Has Alzheimer's Disease
Jake is employed as a teacher. He is the father of two children and describes himself as happily married. His mother recently moved in with his family because she was unable to live independently in her home due to progression of Alzheimer's disease. He stated feeling fearful that his mother would soon not recognize him or her grandchildren. He stated that he is not sleeping at night because he is afraid his mother may try to leave the house, even though he has placed precautions throughout the house, such as extra door locks, cameras, alarms, and motion detectors. Jake said his sleep problems began about one year ago, when his mother was diagnosed with rapid onset of Alzheimer's disease.

He has a history of high blood pressure and was slightly overweight for his age, gender, and height. Other than taken blood pressure medication, his medical history is nonsignificant. He denies recreational drugs and drinks alcohol in social situations. He goes to bed at 8:30 p.m. but does not fall asleep until 11:30 p.m. Jake turns on the television and watches his favorites evening shows. He is unable to fall asleep until after the news. He stated that he has two or three nocturnal awakenings with the need to urinate and is unable to return to sleep immediately. He will check on his mother and children and check to make sure all the doors are locked and the alarm is set, and then he will go back to bed. Jake stated that he will turn on his bedside lamp and read a mystery novel (he really enjoys mystery novels) and will fall asleep within one or two hours. Jake was given a sleep diary. He agreed to complete the log and return it during his next visit.

Jake presented for his second appointment, and his sleep log was reviewed. Jake drinks one or two cups of coffee in the early morning and eats dinner at around 7:00 p.m. His sleep log is reflective of what he initially stated was his bedtime, the actual time that he falls asleep, and time to return to sleep after a nocturnal awakening. Jake was instructed to not go to his bedroom until 11:30 p.m., and he is to stop watching television at 10:00 p.m. and engage in calming, relaxing behaviors. Jake initially pushed back and stated that his bedroom was relaxing, and he did not understand why he could not watch television in bed. When asked if stayed up to watch the evening news, he stated that he looks forward to the news and wants to keep current on city, state, and national events. Stimulus control techniques and sleep hygiene behaviors were explained, along with helpful sleep-promoting behaviors versus sleep activities that negatively impact sleep.

He was told not to read at night because he enjoys reading and it is a mentally stimulating activity for him. Jake stated that reading is his way of unwinding and taking his mind off things, including worrying about his mother—it is his down time. He was asked what activities he enjoys that are not mentally stimulating, but he was unable to report any behavior other than watching television and/or reading as relaxing. He was asked if he was familiar with deep breathing and relaxation techniques; he stated that he had an audio tape on relaxation with guided imagery. He was instructed to put the audio tape on after the evening news, listen to the audio tape in any room but his bedroom, and return to his bed only when he felt sleepy. Stimulus control techniques were utilized so that he would learn to associate his bed with sleep (and sexual activities). He agreed to try. Last, he was instructed to limit his fluid intake during the evening hours to help reduce his nocturnal awakening associated with going to the bathroom.

At appointment three, Jake stated that he was unable to avoid reading at nighttime. He described feeling anxious when he tried to listen to the audio tapes because he was worried about his mother. CBT techniques were utilized to challenge his faulty beliefs that watching television and reading would somehow be protective behaviors regarding his mother. He was able to discern that watching television and reading was a distraction, and he did not check his mother's room monitors because he knew that the house and his mother were safe. Jake made the connection that deep breathing and guided imagery are relaxing; he just had to get used to doing them and to try to not let his mind wander.

At appointment four, Jake stated that the first six days of the week were very difficult and that he spent more time awake than he had prior to coming to the sleep clinic. Review of his sleep log showed that he was getting one hour less sleep than prior to the sleep intervention. Jake described the cause was trying to learn to relax at night to listening to the audio tapes. He stated that he would start to fall asleep and quickly return to his bed, but then he was wide awake and would go back and forth until he felt sleepy enough to fall asleep. Last, his sleep awakenings had declined to one time per night, and he was able to return to sleep.

At appointment five, review of Jake's sleep diary revealed that he was sleeping, on average, 7 hours per night. He only listened to his guided imagery audio tape for about 10–15 minutes and was able to fall asleep in his bed. Jake continued to have one nocturnal awakening due to the need to urinate and was able to return to sleep. Jake stated that instead of meeting for future appointments, he would send his sleep log in, and if he continued with positive sleep behaviors and waking up feeling refreshed, then he would not need to continue with sleep intervention. He agreed to return if his sleep began to deteriorate.

In summary, Jake was able to continue reporting positive progress. He also stated that he joined a caregivers' Alzheimer's group, and it has been very beneficial. He reported decreased anxiety regarding his mother and his ability to have more pleasant interactions with her. Jake reported focusing less on her disease and more on her and her relationship with him and his family.

There is no quick way to "fix" an insomniac's sleep. These scenarios illustrate that the clinician needs to know what types of treatment modalities are to be used to treat sleep disturbance (e.g., decreasing anxiety, changing faulty beliefs, engaging in healthy sleep behaviors, and learning hypnosis/or relaxing behaviors).

References

M. Aldrich (2000). Cardinal manifestations of sleep disorders. In M. H. Kryger, T. Roth, & W. C. Dement (Eds.), *Principles and practice of sleep medicine* (3rd ed., pp. 526–528). Philadelphia, PA: W.B. Saunders Company.

American Psychiatric Association (2013). *Diagnostic and statistical manual of mental disorders* (5th ed.). Arlington, VA: American Psychiatric Publishing.

K. E. Bauer, & T. R. McCanne (1980). An hypnotic technique for treating insomnia. *International Journal of Clinical & Experimental Hypnosis, 28*(1), 1–5.

J. H. Benington (2000). Sleep homeostasis and the function of sleep. *Sleep, 23*(7), 959–966.

P. A. Blissitt (2001). Sleep, memory, and learning. *Journal of Neuroscience Nursing, 33*(4), 208–215.

J. Born, T. Lange, K. Hansen, M. Molle, & H. L. Fehm (1997). Effects of sleep and circadian rhythm on human circulating immune cells. *Journal of Immunology, 158*(9), 4454–4464.

W. C. Dement, & C. Vaughan (2000). *The promise of sleep*. New York: Random House, Inc.

J. D. Edinger, W. K. Wohlgemuth, R. A. Radtke, G. R. Marsh, & R. E. Quillian (2001). Cognitive behavioral therapy for treatment of chronic primary insomnia: A randomized controlled trial. *JAMA: Journal of the American Medical Association, 285*(14), 1856–1864.

B. Ehrenberg (2000). Importance of sleep restoration in co-morbid disease: Effect of anticonvulsants. *Neurology, 54*(5 Suppl. 1), S33–37.

G. Graci, & J. Hardie (2007). Evidenced based hypnotherapy for the management of sleep disorder. *International Journal of Clinical and Experimental Hypnosis, 55*(3), 288–302.

G. Graci, & K. Sexton-Radek (2005). Treatment of sleep disorders using hypnosis and cognitive-behavioral therapies. In R. Chapman (Ed.) *A practitioner's case book on CBT and Hypnosis* (pp. 349–359). New York: Springer Publications Company.

D. Hammond (1990). Sleep disorders. In D. Hammond (Ed.), *Handbook of hypnotic suggestions and metaphors* (pp. 220–221). New York: W.W. Norton & Company, Inc.

P. J. Hauri (1993). Consulting about insomnia: A method and some preliminary data. *Sleep: Journal of Sleep Research & Sleep Medicine, 16*(4), 344–350.

P. J. Hauri (2000). The many faces of insomnia. In D. I. Mostofsky & D. H. Barlow (Eds.), *The management of stress and anxiety in medical disorders* (pp. 143–159). Needham Heights, MA: Allyn & Bacon.

L. A. Hodgson (1991). Why do we need sleep? Relating theory to nursing practice. *Journal of Advanced Nursing, 16*(12), 1503–1510.

J. Krueger, & F. Obal (1993). A neuronal group theory of sleep function. *Journal of Sleep Research, 2*(2), 63–69.

M. Kryger (2004). *A woman's guide to sleep disorders* (1st ed.). New York: McGraw-Hill.

M. Kryger, T. Roth, & W. C. Dement (2001). Principles and practice of sleep medicine. *Depression & Anxiety, 13*(3), 157.

L. Lamberg (2000). Sleep disorders, often unrecognized, complicate many physical illnesses. *JAMA, 284*(17), 2173–2175.

K. A. Lee (1997). An overview of sleep and common sleep problems. *ANNA Journal, 24*, 614–623.

R. Manber, & T. Kuo (2002). Cognitive-behavioral therapies for insomnia. In T. L. Lee-Chiong, M. J. Satela, M. A. Carskadon, & M. A. Carskadon (Eds.), *Sleep medicine* (pp. 177–185). Philadelphia, PA: Hanley and Belfus Inc.

P. Maquet (2001). The role of sleep in learning and memory. *Science, 294*(5544), 1048–1052.

M. Mills & G. Graci (2004). Sleep disturbances. In M. Frogge (Ed.), *Cancer symptom management* (pp. 111–134). Sudbury, MA: Jones & Bartlett Publishers.

T. Modlin (2002). Sleep disorders and hypnosis: To cope or cure? *Sleep & Hypnosis, 4*(1), 39–46.

C. M. Morin (1993). *Insomnia: Psychological assessment and management*. New York: Guilford Press.

C. M. Morin (1999a). "Behavioral and pharmacological treatment for insomnia": Reply. *JAMA: Journal of the American Medical Association, 282*(12), 1130–1131.

C. M. Morin. (1999b). Empirically supported psychological treatments: A natural extension of the scientist-practitioner paradigm. *Canadian Psychology, 40*(4), 312–315.

C. M. Morin. (2000). The nature of insomnia and the need to refine our diagnostic criteria. *Psychosomatic Medicine, 62*(4), 483–485.

C. M. Morin (2003). Measuring outcomes in randomized clinical trials of insomnia treatments. *Sleep Medicine Reviews, 7*(3), 263–279.

C. M. Morin (2004). Insomnia treatment: Taking a broader perspective on efficacy and cost-effectiveness issues. *Sleep Medicine Reviews, 8*(1), 3–6.

C. M. Morin, & N. H. Azrin (1987). Stimulus control and imagery training in treating sleep-maintenance insomnia. *Journal of Consulting & Clinical Psychology, 55*(2), 260–262.

C. M Morin, & N. H. Azrin, (1988). Behavioral and cognitive treatments of geriatric insomnia. *Journal of Consulting and Clinical Psychology, 56*(5), 748–753.

C. M. Morin, C. Bastien, & J. Savard (2003). Current status of cognitive-behavior therapy for insomnia: Evidence for treatment effectiveness and feasibility. In M. L. Perlis & K. L. Lichstein (Eds.), *Treating sleep disorders: Principles and practice of behavioral sleep medicine* (pp. 262–285). New York: John Wiley & Sons, Inc.

C. M. Morin, & J. Ware (1996). Sleep and psychopathology. *Applied & Preventive Psychology, 5*(4), 211–224.

National Sleep Foundation (2017). *What causes insomnia?* Retrieved January 17, 2019, from https://sleepfoundation.org/insomnia/content/what-causes-insomnia

M. J. Sateia (2014). International Classification of Sleep Disorders-Third Edition: Highlights and Modifications. *Chest, 146*(5), 1387–1394. https://doi.org/10.1378/chest.14-0970.

M. J. Sateia, K. Doghramji, P. J. Hauri, & C. M. Morin (2000). Evaluation of chronic insomnia. An American Academy of Sleep Medicine review. *Sleep, 23*(2), 243–308.

J. Savard, S. M. Miller, M. Mills, A. O'Leary, H. Harding, S. D. Douglas, et al. (1999). Association between subjective sleep quality and depression on immunocompetence in low-income women at risk for cervical cancer. *Psychosomatic Medicine, 61*(4), 496–507.

J. Savard, & C. M. Morin (2001). Insomnia in the context of cancer: a review of a neglected problem. *Journal of Clinical Oncology, 19*(3), 895–908.

J. Savard, S. Simard, J. Blanchet, H. Ivers, & C. M. Morin (2001). Prevalence, clinical characteristics, and risk factors for insomnia in the context of breast cancer. *Sleep, 24*(5), 583–590.

T. J. Sejnowski, & A. Destexhe (2000). Why do we sleep? *Brain Research, 886*(1–2), 208–223.

K. Sexton-Radek, & G. Graci (2008). *Combating sleep disorders.* Santa Barbara, CA: Praeger.

J. M. Siegel (2001). The REM sleep-memory consolidation hypothesis. *Science, 294*(5544), 1058–1063.

A. Spielman & M. W. Anderson (2004). Assessment and differential diagnosis of insomnia. In *Insomnia.* Boston, MA: Springer.

A. Weitzenhoffer (2000). The induction of hypnosis. In *The practice of hypnotism.* New York: John Wiley & Sons.

J. Wilson-Barnett, L. Batehup, & M. Fordam (1988). *Patient problems: A research base for nursing care.* London: Scutari Press.

CHAPTER 2

Sleep Apnea

Sleep apnea is characterized by loud snoring, irritableness, and daytime sleepiness. Cessation of breathing and loud snoring can also be quite problematic to the sleeper's bed partner. In fact, the physiological components of these characteristics make it a profoundly serious medical condition. Furthermore, current public health studies identified an increase in sleep apnea.

There are two classifications of sleep apnea: central and obstructive. Obstructive sleep apnea (OSA) is more common and is the focus of this chapter. It is defined as the cessation or partial cessation of airflow, accompanied by pressure on respiratory drive. If there is a partial reduction in oxygen, it is called a hypopnea.

The all-night polysomnogram is essential to OSA diagnoses. The sleep technician examines the information from the sensors placed on the patient's body about their brainwave patterns, heart rate, breathing, muscle tone of their chin and thigh muscle and eye movements. The Sleep Medicine scoring procedure systematically classifies each type of measurement into sleep behaviors. With Sleep Apnea scoring rules during a sleep study are set up to indicate the patient stops breathing and during which stage of sleep. Some overnight studies are repeated once the sleep pattern is determined with the plan to start the continuous positive air pressure (CPAP) device during the sleep study to determine how it works for the patients and to determine the optimal setting for the CPAP. The CPAP looks like a small plastic mask that has a small hose attached to it that the patient wears. Under the supervision of the board-certified sleep specialist, the overnight study is examined with specialized software that they use to determine if apnea occurred, how severe it was, and what stage of sleep the apnea occurred. The breathing cessation event and reduction in oxygen levels are reflected in the apnea hypopnea index (AHI). The severity of OSA is indicated by the AHI. Furthermore, the AHI has been found to be associated with severity of disease (i.e., cardiovascular, endocrine, neurocognitive).

The Scope of OSA

The incidence of OSA is 3–7% of adults and 1–4% of children in the United States. The gender ratio is 1:2 females to males with OSA. OSA is reduced across the life span. With advancing age, more males, particularly Black and Asian males, have a higher rate of OSA. OSA incidence increases with body mass index increases. Additionally, the presence of OSA increases the risk of developing cardiovascular disease, congestive heart failure, polycystic ovary syndrome, and asthma.

The reader is directed to Pressman and Orr (1996) for a specific discussion of causative factors related to OSA. Briefly stated, imbalances in upper airway pressure, ventilation and oxygenation responses in the upper airway, upper airway recruitment of alternate musculature, and intra-esophageal pressure response to arousal are considered the core elements necessary for patent airway. Anatomical and physiological conditions that influence these factors place the individual at greater risk of OSA. Most recent research focus has been on the association between obesity and OSA. Increased weight compresses the upper airway structures thought to be responsible for OSA. Increased testosterone in men and androgen levels in postmenopausal women have been identified as influential factors to OSA. The changes in these factors must coincide with other respiratory events, such as diaphragmatic movements.

In young children, allergy and asthma, nasopharyngeal factors, and enlarged adenoids have been identified as risk factors. Increasing basic metabolic panels (BMPs) in children complicates the current circumstances of childhood obesity and sleep apnea. In some cases, facial tissue and bone structure are significant factors precipitating OSA. The myriad of factors related to the development of OSA creates varied patient presentations.

A sleep specialist will conduct a physical exam, with notation of the patient's neck circumference, tonsil size, nasal obstruction, uvular prominence, pharyngeal tissue size, craniofacial features, and palate position. Following this, an all-night polysomnographic recording of the patient's sleep will be conducted. If the patient is a child, additional craniofacial measurements would be made. The American Association of Sleep Medicine (AASM) has generated a sleep study protocol and validity comparison mechanism to compare children with sleep disordered breathing to age-matched controls. Importantly, if the apnea and hypopnea begin during the sleep study, the AASM has a distinct protocol that must be followed. The protocol includes the positioning of a continuous positive airway pressure mask on the patient. In minor apnea or hypopnea cases, changing one's sleep position may be the only treatment needed.

Central sleep apnea is characterized by a particular breathing pattern. Central sleep apnea is less common than OSA, and it does not respond to continuous positive airway pressure (CPAP) as successfully as OSA does. Other breathing related disorders are upper airway resistance syndrome, obesity-hypoventilation syndrome, and congenital central hypoventilation syndrome.

OSA patients present with daytime sleepiness and mood irritability and commonly have large body habitus, where their neck circumference is greater than 17 inches. Questions that address these factors are often asked as part of physical exams and for presurgical evaluations. In more chronic manifestations, patients will present with mental health issues of depression.

An apnea is defined as a reduction of airflow by 90% for 10 seconds. The number of apnea events per hour are noted during a nighttime polysomnogram (PSG), and then categorized into mild, moderate, or severe levels. When the body mass index (BMI) exceeds 39, the amount of body fat, including that in the pharynx and larynx areas, is relaxed or compressed, thus closing the breath aperture. Although infrequent in lean people, OSA can occur due to flaccid muscle in the throat causing the same outcome—lack of structure integrity within the throat and consequential collapsing of tissue and a closing of the aperture.

Sleep research studies have identified the cognitive consequences of OSA (Sexton-Radek, 2013). Over time, the quality of cognitive performance decreases with difficulty sustaining attention, the level and amount of divergent thinking, high distractibility, and difficulty encoding into short-term memory. These significant cognitive impairments lead to substantial social functioning decrements.

The metabolic effects of untreated OSA result in an impaired insulin secretion response to glucose and decreased insulin effectiveness in stimulating glucose uptake by skeletal muscle and in restraining hepatic glucose production. If these difficulties are untreated, the individual with OSA is at risk for metabolic syndrome.

Meslier et al. (2003) recorded decreases in insulin sensitivity in a sample of 595 patients, of which 494 were diagnosed. All scored in the moderate to severe range [apnea hypopnea index (AHd) >10]. The insulin resistance occurs and is complicated by the release of proinflammatory cytokines that affect metabolism. In a study of severe OSA patients, Harsch et al. (2004) identified that patients with an apnea hypopnea index of greater than 20 had dose response increases in insulin sensitivity as they used the CPAP machine.

Two epidemiological studies, the Wisconsin Sleep Cohort Study and the Sleep Heart Health Study, documented the increased risk for development of hypertension in patients with OSA. Both studies reported these findings, regardless of the age, gender, ethnicity, and BMI of the participants.

With each apnea episode, an increase in heart rate and blood pressure occur at the termination of the apnea that is thought to be driven by the hypoxia (decrease in circulating oxygen). It is believed that the heart rate and blood pressure increases of the apneas in the untreated OSA patient promulgate increased sympathetic tone and activation of the Renin-Angiotensin system (Mansukhani, Kara, Caples, & Somers, 2014). The cardiovascular drain associated with untreated OSA is related to the sustained sympathetic tone. Specifically, heightened sympathetic activates leading to vasoconstriction, tachycardia, and increased catechol. OSA is directly implicated in cardiovascular distress.

Rogers (2003) has summarized the number of studies of individuals with chronic sleep loss. A subgroup of this population is untreated OSA patients. Overall, neurobehavior deficits of cognitive functioning decline and maladaptive social functioning increases at a steady rate from day three of sleep loss/poor sleep onward.

OSA and Other Sleep Factors

In their analysis of sleep patients with insomnia, OSA, and Periodic Limb Movement (PLM) disorder diagnoses, Vanable, Aikins, Tadineti, Caruana-Montaldo, and Mendelson (2000) identified that participants complained of poor sleep quality more so if the time after a wake up was increasing through the night. That is, in addition to the objective findings of the consequences of poor sleep in OSA patients, a perceptual component of subjective poor sleep influences their sleepiness in the day. Yo-El et al. (2016) determined the levels of derived proteins in cerebrospinal fluid distinguish OSA patients from Alzheimer's patients and controls. The recurrent arousals and hypoxia were determining factors in the decrease of amyloid and neuronally derived proteins in Cerebral Spinal Fluid (CSF). Sexton-Radek (2013) identified the positive correlation of increases in respiratory effort and measured levels of blood pressure in an untreated OSA patient. The study was conducted in the interval between a PSG diagnosis and delivery of a CPAP machine, with follow-ups extending to three months.

Medical Status of the Consequences of OSA

Canessa et al. (2014) designed an OSA trial investigating the impairments in reported daytime sleepiness and cognitive function declines in untreated OSA patients. The repetitive hypoxia was particularly toxic to the entorhinal cortex areas of the hippocampus, left posterior parietal cortex, and right superior frontal gyrus in untreated OSA patients. Because of this danger to patients, presurgical screening protocols have been designed to detect OSA. The STOP-Bang questionnaire is a screening tool commonly used by surgeons and physicians to detect OSA. Dimitrou and Macavei (2016) reviewed the usage pattern of the STOP-Bang questionnaire and other prescreening scales. They concluded that the STOP-Bang questionnaire is helpful in determining perioperative and postoperative complications (i.e., including OSA) in patients. Additional research in this area has identified the validity and utility of the STOP-Bang questionnaire in the detection of OSA and other perisurgical/postsurgical complications (Chung & Elsaid, 2009; Nagappa, Won, Singh, Wong, & Chung, 2017; Nagappa et al., 2015).

Additional medical studies to identify OSA have been with the use of a oximeter. The application of an oximeter, where oxygen desaturation patterns are used to extrapolate sleep parameters, are commonly used (Bohning et al., 2010). A review of oximeter use indicated that it was adequate for a hospital population in a home setting to detect difficulty. However, the oximeter is not adequate to diagnose OSA (Collop et al., 2011).

Diagnosis and Treatment of OSA

A CPAP provided by a mask administering airflow provides a pneumatic stent to the atrophied or cellular missignaled tissue of the OSA patient. CPAP devices, since 1980, have provided millions of patients with enriched sleep quality and reduced cardiovascular and metabolic complications from the apneic events. Huntley, Kaffenberger, Doghramiji,

Soose, and Boon (2017) reported significant improvement in OSA patients in terms of reduced postoperative AHd. Ravesloot, White, Heinper, Oksenberg, and Pepin (2017) identified the utility of positional devices in OSA patients with a mild range AHd. The custom fit and variable settings of the CPAP device not only contribute to the patient control and compliance but also provide a means for the sleep specialists to prescribe the intensity of the treatment (Johal, Haria, Manek, Joury, & Rija, 2017).

Home PSG studies provide a convenience to the patient and a measure that may not otherwise be obtained to the sleep specialist. However, controversy exists among the experts, with a substantiated consensus that oximetry underestimates sleep apnea severity (Bianchi & Goparaju, 2017; Setty, 2017). Newer measurement values such as ocular changes and ratings of degree of ptosis are of current research and clinical consideration (Santos & Hofmann, 2017). Last, neuroimaging studies validate the cardiovascular changes and resultant reduction in gray matter density of chronic OSA patients (Yaouhi et al., 2009; Zimmerman & Aloia, 2006).

Additional Treatment

Inspire Therapy

For patients who are intolerant to CPAP, there is an alternative called inspire therapy (Strollo et al., 2014), which was Food and Drug Administration (FDA) approved in 2012. Inspire therapy is a small device that is inserted during an outpatient surgery, restoring muscle tone to a patient's airway (Professionals, 2019). The patient's airway is controlled using a remote-control device and is monitored using a cloud-based adherence system.

Eligibility requirements are based on the following: moderate to severe OSA, unable to achieve consistent benefit from CPAP, patients are not significantly overweight, and patients are age 22 or older. Inspire therapy has shown improvements in daytime sleepiness, restoration of altered breathing events during sleep, and reduced loud snoring.

Oral Appliances

Oral appliances (mouth guards) have been successful in treating mild to moderate cases of OSA. Dental professionals can specialize in the treatment of OSA patients with oral appliances. Oral appliances can hold the tongue in place and can ease the jaw forward, creating airway space; this change can reduce the upper airway collapse commonly seen in OSA patients because the mandible is advanced (Sutherland, Vanderveken, Tsuda, Marklund, & Gagnadoux 2014).

Oral appliances require a visit to the dentist for adjustments. They can have varying design features. For instance, pending the anatomy of a patient's mouth and the degree of upper airway collapse, a patient may have a choice between a one-piece mouth guard and a two-piece mouth guard, with separated upper and lower plates (Sutherland et al., 2014).

Patients commonly experience adverse events, including but not limited to mouth dryness, tooth pain, excessive salivation, headaches, and jaw discomfort (Ferguson, Cartwright, Rogers, Schmidt-Nowara, 2006). The side effects of the oral appliance generally last a couple of months; however, pain can last up to 12 months. The primary reasons for oral appliance discontinuation tend to be related to mouth dryness, tooth pain, and/or jaw discomfort. Overall, treatment success is variable—some patients cannot tolerate the oral appliance, because they find it uncomfortable or it is not efficacious.

Oral Surgery

Surgical management of OSA is accomplished by a procedure called uvulopalatopharyngoplasty (UPPP). For those selecting UPPP, genetics may play a large factor in the causation of sleep apnea (Mehra & Wolford, 2000). For instance, having large tonsils, excessive throat tissue, or involvement of the tongue and/or jaw may generate disordered breathing while asleep. For individuals with this type of oral anatomy, UPPP may be a successful alternative to CPAP because the procedure increases the oropharyngeal air space by resecting tissue in the throat, including the uvula, soft palate, and tonsils (Adil & McGinn, 2017).

The adverse events noted with UPPP procedures include having a sore throat lasting several weeks, often requiring pain medication, and pain from stitches in the back of the throat (Icahn School of Medicine at Mount Sinai, 2020). Patients are instructed to eat soft foods and liquids, avoid chewy or crunchy foods, and avoid heavy lifting for the first two weeks postsurgery.

The success rate of UPPP is varied in the literature, ranging from 80% to 40% (Adil & McGinn, 2017). Other researchers suggest that OSA improves initially (about 50%) for those having the UPPP; however, over time, the benefits significantly decline for many patients (Icahn School of Medicine at Mount Sinai, 2020). These researchers suggest that having a UPPP may be best suited for patients who have structural mouth abnormalities.

Weight Loss

The majority of the research suggests that losing weight will significantly improve OSA; however, there is no guarantee that weight reduction will eliminate it. Overweight individuals tend to have thicker necks with extra tissue in the throat, leading to blocks in airway space (AASM, 2020). Many studies illustrate that losing 10% of weight will help improve OSA (Adil & McGinn, 2017; American Thoracic Society, 2009). CPAP compliance combined with weight loss strategies are effective in improving OSA.

While there are numerous CPAP treatments, this chapter illustrates that surgery may not last. CPAP is only effective if patients adhere to using their CPAP machines consistently (even during daytime napping), and it is a costly device. The one treatment avenue that many patients are reluctant to consider is making permanent lifestyle changes aimed at weight reduction. Weight loss can "cure" OSA for some but not all patients, especially if there are no structural oral abnormalities present, yet patients are reluctant—or refuse—to go down the weight-loss path.

The challenges reported by patients are finding the time to exercise, not enjoying exercise (including that it is too difficult or that they do not want to do it alone), not knowing the right types of foods to eat, limiting food intake, and not wanting to commit to making lifestyle changes. These reported challenges can be addressed by finding a buddy or partner to exercise with, joining an exercise group or fitness club, participating in low-impact exercise, taking it slowly (no one is expected to complete a marathon), going to a nutritionist, working out from home, and understanding the long-term benefits of weight reduction (e.g., reduced blood pressure, improved cardiac function, improvements in joint pain).

Positional Therapy

Patients who experience mild to moderate OSA while sleeping in the supine (back) position are more likely to have apneic events and reported sleep disturbance (Ravesloot, van Maanen, Dun, & de Vries, 2013). If the OSA events do not occur during REM/deep sleep, positional therapy will be successful. The most common and very inexpensive way to improve OSA for those with mild to moderate OSA is to have patients learn to *not* sleep on their backs. Essentially, the clinician teaches patients to become side sleepers. There are devices on the market that attach to your waist or back to eliminate back sleeping. Positional therapy can be used alone or with CPAP to treat OSA.

The T-shirt method is a common method that involves sewing a pocket on the back of a T-shirt and inserting a tennis ball in it. If patients fall asleep on their sides, and then move to the supine position during sleep, they will immediately wake up because the tennis ball is pressing into their backs. Over time, patients become conditioned to not sleep on their backs. This method also helps those who snore loudly when sleeping in the supine position.

CPAP Treatment Summary

In summary, the gold standard treatment for OSA is to use CPAP, which increases the pharyngeal airway space during sleep. CPAP use can also be combined with weight reduction strategies and positional therapy. It is important for patients to continue to follow up with their sleep clinicians because if there is weight reduction, the CPAP pressure may need to be reevaluated. The challenges to CPAP include patient acceptance, tolerance, and compliance because these challenges often reduce effectiveness (Sutherland et al., 2014). If patients are not compliant with CPAP use, the OSA symptoms immediately return, reducing quality of life, mental awareness, energy, and so on. It is important to use CPAP even when napping during the daytime. With the evolution of CPAP devices, the current machines are quieter and much smaller than previous ones. Patients should not be reluctant to purchase CPAP equipment because the machines are travel friendly and are relatively lightweight. Use of CPAP as stated not only improves lives but reduces the chances of work injuries, automobile accidents, and other instances related to safety.

Effects and Costs

In Society

A recent publication by Breus (2013) identified the phenomena of "sleep divorce." There is increasing number of couples, estimated to be 25% in the United States, who are sleeping apart. It is believed that this number is on the rise. Different schedules, disrupted sleep of one partner in the couple, conflicts with cosleeping (child, pet), poor sleep.environment, and divergent sleep habits have been identified as factors contributing to "sleep divorces" in the United States.

In Relationships

In 2006, Dr. Rosalind Cartwright of the Sleep Disorder Center at Rush University Medical Center in Chicago, Illinois, conducted a scientific study to evaluate how a husband's sleep apnea impacts the wife's quality of sleep and the couple's marital satisfaction. The findings from the Married Couples Sleep Study of ten couples identified extreme sleep deprivation in the wives due to the noisy gasping for air and snoring associated with their husbands' OSA. Once they slept alone, the wives' scores on marital satisfaction and sleep quality increased.

For some mild cases of OSA, a change in the sleep position to either side or stomach is helpful in stopping the snoring. In this area, several creative inventions (such as Dr. Cartwright's T-shirt with a back pocket for tennis balls) provide a deterrent to sleeping on one's back, a position that is conducive to snoring.

With treatment for husbands with OSA, marital satisfaction increased. It seems that this synchronization of a couple's sleep is positively associated with marital satisfaction as well.

At Work

The work impairment index showing absenteeism/presenteeism indicated that sleep and work impairment are correlated. When sleep duration drops below six hours nightly, the values of absenteeism/presenteeism increase. In undiagnosed OSA, sleep is abbreviated and fragmented. Workplace productivity, as measured by work lost secondary to absenteeism/presenteeism, is important to address. Work lost to absenteeism or from productivity in the United States was estimated to be 1,234,814 days per year based on the National Sleep Foundation Census Survey (National Sleep Foundation, 2013).

Case Study 1

Bernie was referred the sleep clinic by a gastric bypass clinic to get him on CPAP and the appropriate pressure for the surgery. He was on a medical leave from work due to incidences of falling asleep at the wheel while driving a bus. Bernie was a 36-year-old male city bus driver who was morbidly obese and had a history of high blood pressure. He denied any additional medical issues; he also denied snoring, nocturnal leg movements, or difficulty falling asleep or staying asleep. Bernie did not have a bed partner to confirm his sleep history.

Bernie endorsed using recreational drugs and alcohol once to twice per week (usually on weekends). He discussed falling asleep for one to two hours when he arrived home from work, and would eat dinner and doze off while watching television. He did not wake up feeling refreshed. He stated that he often fell asleep during the day, especially during his lunch hour. Last, Bernie stated that he dozed off while watching television, at the movies, and occasionally while eating dinner. He also stated that he would doze off sometimes when using the restroom. He denied injuring himself when dozing off.

He was administered the Epworth Sleepiness Scale (Johns, 1991) and scored greater than 16 indicating that he had very high chances of dozing off in all types of situations.

Bernie stated that he needed to lose weight to return to work. When asked what his weight loss strategies had been, he stated that he did not want to exercise (did not like to), had never worked with a nutritionist, and had no interest in trying to lose weight by changing his eating habits. He understood that he would need to change the quantity of food intake and the quality of his food once he had the gastric bypass surgery. He stated that he just needed to lose weight quickly so that he could return to work.

Bernie was scheduled for an overnight polysomnogram and daytime sleep study. His apnea index was significant high, meaning there were many times during the nighttime sleep period that he stopped breathing and had an arousal (woke up) to start the breathing process again. During the nighttime sleep study, Bernie was placed on CPAP and was able to significantly restore his sleep and significantly improve his sleep-disordered breathing.

Bernie was prescribed a CPAP machine and the appropriate CPAP pressure settings. His surgeon was sent this information so that he could be treated during surgery with the correct CPAP pressure settings. Bernie was scheduled to return for a follow-up visit. He did not return and was lost to follow-up.

Case Study 2

Enzo presented to the sleep clinic due to complaints of daytime sleepiness and having difficulty with work performance. Enzo owned a cabinet and flooring company and not only ran the business but managed more than 40 workers. He stated that he had fallen asleep at the wheel while waiting at a stoplight, at his desk, while watching television, while eating dinner, and any time that does not require paying attention to details or when he is not engaged in activities requiring vigilance.

Enzo was a 52-year-old male who was six foot two inches tall and weighed 325 pounds. He was overweight and had a neck circumference of 18 inches. He reported going to bed at around 11:00 pm and waking up at 6:30 a.m. and that he did not feel refreshed upon awakening. He had to set three alarms to get him out of bed by 6:45 a.m. He denied snoring, nocturnal leg movements, or difficulty falling asleep or maintaining sleep. He indicated that he got up one or two times per night to urinate but fell back to sleep without incidence. He did not have a bed partner. He scored significant daytime sleepiness on his Epworth Sleep Scale test.

Enzo was scheduled for a multiple sleep latency test (MSLT) to determine the extent of his daytime sleepiness and a nocturnal PSG to determine his level of nocturnal sleep quality and extent of daytime sleepiness. Results of his MSLT revealed that he had extensive daytime sleepiness. His PSG revealed that he had significant OSA events. He was treated with CPAP during the PSG and reached an effective CPAP pressure to reduce the number of apneic events. His apneic events occurred in all sleeping positions.

Enzo was prescribed a CPAP machine and was asked to return for follow-up appointments to determine his level of compliance. Enzo returned for all follow-up visits, and a review of his CPAP usage showed that he was compliant and that the compliance continued over the course of one year. Enzo reported that when he forgot to use his CPAP machine, he immediately noticed the return of daytime sleepiness and difficulty with focusing on work-related tasks.

Enzo started working out at home and changed his eating habits, and he lost 40 pounds over the course of four months. He returned for another nocturnal PSG, and his CPAP pressure was reduced because his weight loss improved his OSA. He again was compliant with his CPAP usage and his follow-up appointments.

Four months later, during a follow-up appointment, he stated that he felt that his CPAP pressure might be too high for him. Enzo reported losing another 30 pounds and returned for a PSG to determine if his CPAP pressure was too high. Results revealed that his continued weight loss further contributed to a reduction in OSA events, and his CPAP pressure was lowered. Over the course of two and a half years, Enzo reduced his weight from 325 to 185 pounds and no longer used CPAP because his OSA was no longer at the clinical level. He reported feeling awake and energetic during the day, and sleeping well at night.

Enzo attributed his success in OSA treatment mainly on his compliance with CPAP because he was able to have the energy and focus to not only function at work but also exercise at home. He stated that he would walk around his neighborhood, doing lunges and stomach crunches and using free weights to reduce the weight and to improve not only his physical strength but his cardiac functioning. He also worked with a nutritionist to reduce his food intake and to eat smaller, healthier meals. Enzo stated that it took dedication and determination to lose the weight, but CPAP was the key to his success. Enzo keeps in contact with his sleep clinician and states that his commitment to exercise and food lifestyle changes have remained. He also stated that he completed a half marathon at the age of 55.

Case Study 3
Martha was a 26-year-old female who was 5 foot 3 inches tall and weighed 118 pounds. Her neck was 14 inches in circumference. She worked in her family's restaurant assisting with early morning food preparation and serving customers during dining hours. She presented to the sleep clinic with complaints of loud snoring and feeling sleepy during the day. She stated that she fell asleep while chopping vegetables at work and received eight stitches to her hand. She also confirmed falling asleep while watching television and has had to pull over when driving due to sleepiness.

She denied complaints of nocturnal leg movements, difficulty falling or staying asleep, or having any REM or NREM sleep issues. She stated that she went to bed at 1:00 a.m. and woke up at 9:00 a.m. and did not feel refreshed upon awakening. She often turned the alarm off to get more sleep. She often arrived at her family's restaurant late, and this tardiness created tension with her family because they do not seem to understand the extent of her sleepiness.

Results of her Epworth Sleep Score revealed that she was moderately to significantly sleepy during the day. She was scheduled for a daytime MSLT and nocturnal PSG. Her MSLT revealed that she slept during the daytime but had disrupted sleep. Her PSG results showed that she had moderate OSA, and with CPAP, she was able to restore her sleep and eliminated OSA events.

When she returned for her sleep test results, she stated that she did not want to use CPAP because she did not want to be "tied to a machine." She also stated that she researched the side effects of CPAP and decided that it was not an option. She asked about the use of oral appliances and was explained how they function and how they can improve OSA. She was given the name of a dentist who specialized in the creation of oral appliances, and she stated that she would schedule an appointment.

Martha contacted her sleep clinician and requested a follow-up appointment because her oral appliance was painful and the side effects, such as dry mouth, were too much. Her tooth and jaw pain are significant, and she did not want to continue to experience the pain in moving her jaw.

During her appointment, she wanted to discuss other options for OSA treatment. She stated that she was feeling more energetic during the day and was waking up slightly more refreshed. The pros and cons of surgery procedures, such as oral surgery and inspire therapy, were discussed. She declined these options because she did not want to have surgery. Her OSA was not related to position, and she did not need to lose weight because her body habitus was slender.

CPAP was reintroduced, focusing on the benefits and the types of machines that are small and can easily be packed for travel. Different types of facial and nasal masks were shown to her. Martha stated that she would like to try CPAP. She was prescribed CPAP and was asked to return to the clinic in two weeks.

When Martha returned to the clinic, her compliance was 85%, and she stated that CPAP has made a noticeable difference in both her energy and mood. She stated that her compliance was not 100% because of times when she arrived home from work so late that she fell asleep on the couch.

Her third-month follow-up revealed that Martha's main complaint was that her nasal mask was uncomfortable, yet her compliance was 90%. She was fitted with a different type of face mask, and her compliance rate improved to 98%. She no longer took off her nasal mask because it was uncomfortable during sleep. Martha reported an additional increase in mood, energy, focus at work, and overall quality of life.

She had not fallen asleep during work or when driving or watching television. She brought her CPAP machine into the living room and put her face mask on when she was watching television so that if she fell asleep, her sleep would not be affected by apneic events. Martha stated that her only "regret" is that she did not start CPAP when she was first diagnosed with OSA.

Case Study 4

Yvette was a 47-year-old female construction worker with complaints of daytime sleepiness. She had difficulty concentrating during the day and did not wake up feeling refreshed. She denied any work-related accidents. Yvette was five foot seven inches and weighed 130 pounds with a slender build. Her neck circumference was 15 inches. She had a bed partner who reported loud snoring but did not notice moments when she stopped breathing.

She presented to the sleep clinic because she fell asleep at the wheel when stopped at a stoplight, her foot slipped off the brake, and her car hit the car in front of her. Her general practitioner referred her to the sleep clinic to evaluate her for OSA. Results of the Epworth Sleepiness Scale test showed that she was moderately sleepy during the day. She was scheduled for a MSLT and PSG.

Results of her MSLT test showed moderate daytime sleepiness, and her PSG test revealed that she had moderate OSA, combined with snoring. The snoring did cause awakenings. CPAP was used during the sleep test, and an effective CPAP pressure was identified. She was also found to have positional OSA, with most of the apneic events occurring in the supine position.

Yvette stated that she did not want to try CPAP because she often traveled and did not want to have to carry additional equipment, even though she was educated about the size of CPAP machines. Instead, Yvette wanted to explore oral appliances. She was provided with a referral to a dentist in her area who specialized in the creation of oral appliances for OSA treatment. She wanted to know more about how to treat her OSA with positional therapy. She was provided with positional therapy information and purchased a tennis ball T-shirt at checkout. She was asked to call the sleep center in one week to provide follow-up information on how the T-shirt was working.

She stated that it took a couple of nights to try to get used to the T-shirt; after the third night, she reported that as she started to turn toward the supine position in her sleep, she momentarily woke up and turned back to her side. She reported a slight improvement in daytime alertness and waking up feeling refreshed. Yvette stated that she waited to see if the T-shirt method for OSA treatment would significantly improve her OSA before she scheduled an appointment with the referred dentist.

Yvette reached out to the sleep clinic one month later to provide an OSA treatment update. The dentist told her that she was an excellent candidate for an oral appliance, even though her mouth was very crowded. She received her oral appliance approximately two weeks earlier and stated that her snoring had significantly decreased and she was feeling more alert during the day. Waking up in the morning was still a struggle.

Yvette provided a two-month update and stated that she had to return to the dentist for multiple adjustments but that, overall, she was sleeping better, had more energy during the day, and was waking up feeling refreshed. She also continued to use the tennis ball T-shirt, and her bed partner stated that she was no longer snoring and he was able to sleep through the night without having to go to another room. Her only complaint was mouth dryness, but she was taking an over-the-counter medication to resolve that and some jaw pain, but it has gotten better over time. She still had it but not as bad as when she initially used the mouth guards.

She called to provide an update at the six-month mark. She stated that she continued to have mouth dryness, but the over-the-counter medication seemed to alleviate it, and the jaw pain was 80% better. The combined treatment with the tennis ball T-shirt and oral appliance had significantly improved her quality of life, energy, and work performance. She was recently promoted to a supervisor in her construction job and recently got engaged. Yvette stated that she was very happy that she went with the oral appliance option.

References

AASM (2020, February 1). *Sleep apnea treatments—CPAP*. Sleep Education. Retrieved June 9, 2021, from https://aasm.org/

E. A. Adil, & J. D. McGinn (2017, October 6). *Uvulopalatopharyngoplasty*. Medscape. Retrieved June 9, 2021, from https://reference.medscape.com/

American Thoracic Society (2009, February 9). Losing weight can cure obstructive sleep apnea in overweight patients, study shows. *ScienceDaily*. Retrieved April 21, 2021, from https://www.sciencedaily.com/releases/2009/02/090206081319.htm

M. T. Bianchi, & B. Goparaja (2017). Potential underestimation of sleep apnea severity by at-home kits: Rescoring in-laboratory polysomnography without sleep staging. *Journal of Clinical Sleep Medicine, 13*(4), 551–555.

N. Bohning, B. Schultheier, S. Eilers, T. Penzel, W. Bohning, & E. Schmittendorf (2010). Comparison of pulse oximeters used in sleep medicine for the screening of OSA. *Physiological Measures, 7*, 875–888. https://doi.org/10.1088/0967-3334/317/00

M. Breus (2013). *Have you considered a "sleep divorce."* How to Sleep Better. Retrieved June 9, 2021, from https://thesleepdoctor.com/2013/04/25/have-you-considered-a-sleep-divorce/

N. Canessa, V. Castronovo, S. F. Cappas, M. S. Aloia, S. Marelli, A. Falini, et al. (2014). Obstructive sleep apnea: Brain structural changes and neurocognitive function before and after treatment. *American Journal of Respiratory Critical Care Medicine, 183*, 1419–1426.

F. Chung, & H. Elsaid (2009). Screening for obstructive sleep apnea before surgery, "Why is it important?" *Current opinion in anaesthesiology, 22*, 405–411.

N. A. Collop, S. L. Tracy, V. Kapur, R. Mehra, D. Kuhlen, S. A. Fleishman, & J. M Ojile (2011). Obstructive sleep apnea devices for Out-of-Center

(OOC) testing: Technology evaluation. *Journal of Clinical Sleep Medicine, 7*(3), 531–548.

L. Dimitrou, & V. Macavei (2016). Can screening tolls for obstructive sleep apnea predict post-operative complications? A systematic review of the literature. *Journal of Clinical Sleep Medicine, 12*(9), 1293–1300.

L. J. Epstein, D. Kristo, P. Strollo, N. Friedman, A. Malhotra, S. Patil, et al. (2009). Clinical guidelines for the evaluation, management and long-term care of obstructive sleep apnea in adults. *Journal of Clinical Sleep Medicine, 5*(3), 263–276.

K. A. Ferguson, R. Cartwright, R. Rogers, & W. Schmidt-Nowara (2006). Oral appliances for snoring and obstructive sleep apnea: A review. *Sleep, 29*, 244–262. https://doi.org/10.1093/sleep/29.2.244

I. Harsch, S. Schahin, M. Radespial-Troger, O. Weintz, H. Jahreiss, T. Fuchs, et al. (2004). Continuous positive airway pressure treatment rapidly improves sensitivity in obstructive sleep apnea patients. *American Journal of Respiratory Critical Care Medicine, 169*(2), 156–162.

C. Huntley, T. Kaffenberger, K. Ogham, R. Soose, & M. Boon (2017). Upper airway stimulation for treatment of obstructive sleep apnea: An evaluation and comparison of outcomes at two academic centers. *Journal of Clinical Sleep Medicine, 13*(9), 1075–1079. https://doi.org/10.5664/jcsm.6726

Icahn School of Medicine at Mount Sinai. 2020. *Uvulopalatopharyngoplasty (UPPP)*. Retrieved January 3, 2020, from, https://www.mountsinai.org/health-library/surgery/uvulopalatopharyngoplasty-uppp

Institute of Medicine (2006). *Sleep disorders and sleep deprivation: An Unmet public health problem*. Washington, DC: The National Academies Press. https://doi.org/10.17226/11617

A. Johal, P. Haria, S. Manek, E. Joury, & R. Riha (2017). Ready-made versus custom-made mandibular repositioning devices in sleep apnea: A randomized clinical trial. *Journal of Clinical Sleep Medicine, 13*(2), 175–182.

M. W. Johns (1991). A new method for measuring daytime sleepiness: The Epworth sleepiness scale. *Sleep, 4*(6), 540–545.

M. P. Mansukhani, T. Kara, S. M. Caples, & V. K. Somers (2014). Chemoreflexes, sleep apnea, and sympathetic dysregulation. *Current Hypertension Reports, 16*(9), 476. https://doi.org/10.1007/s11906-014-0476-2

P. Mehra, & L. M. Wolford (2000). Surgical management of obstructive sleep apnea. *Proc (Bayl Univ Med Cent), 13*(4), 338–342.

N. Meslier, F., Gagnadoux, P. Giraud, C. Person, H. Okusu, T. Urban, & J. Racineaux (2003). Impaired glucose-insulin metabolism in males with obstructive sleep apnea. *Journal of European Respiration, 22*(1), 156–160. https://doi.org/10.118310936.03.00089902

M. Nagappa, et al. (2015). Validation of the STOP-Bang Questionnaire as a screening tool for obstructive sleep apnea among different populations: A systematic review and meta-analysis. *PLoS ONE, 10*(12), e0143697. https://doi.org/10.137/journal.pone.0143697

M. Nagappa, P. Liao, J. Wong, D. Auckley, S. Ramachandroan, S. Memtsoudis, et al. (2017). An update on the various practical applications of the STOP-Bang Questionnaire in anesthesia, surgery and perioperative medicine. *Current Opinions in Anesthesiology, 30*, 118–125. https://doi.org/20.1097/ACO.00000000000000.426

National Sleep Foundation (2013). *International bedroom poll summary of findings.* Arlington, VA: National Sleep Foundation.

G. T. O'Connor, B. K. Lind, E. T. Lee, J. Nieto, S. Redline, J. M. Samet, et al. (2002). Variation in symptoms of sleep-disordered breathing with race and ethnicity: The Sleep Heart Health Study. *Sleep, 26*(1), 74–79.

M. R. Pressman, & W. Orr (1997). *Understanding sleep: The evaluation and treatment of sleep disorders.* Washington, DC: American Psychological Association.

M. J. Ravesloot, J. P. van Maanen, L. Dun, & N. de Vries (2013). The undervalued potential of positional therapy in position-dependent snoring and obstructive sleep apnea—a review of the literature. *Sleep Breath, 17*(1), 39–49. https://doi.org/10.1007/s11325-012-0683-5

M. J. Ravesloot, D. White, R. Heinger, A. Oksenberg, & J. Pepin (2017). Efficacy of the new generation of devices for positional therapy for patients with positional obstructive sleep apnea: A systematic review of the literature and meta-analysis. *Journal of Clinical Sleep Medicine, 13*(6), 813–824.

N. L. Rogers (2003). Chronic sleep restriction: Neurobehaioral and endocrine effects. APSS 2003 Post-Graduate Course The Effects of Sleep Loss and Sleep Restriction in Humans, June 3, 2003.

M. Santos, & J. Hofmann (2017). Ocular manifestations of obstructive sleep apnea. *Journal of Clinical Sleep Medicine, 13*(11), 1345–1348.

A. R. Setty (2017). Underestimation of sleep apnea with home sleep apnea testing compared to in-laboratory sleep testing. *Journal of Clinical Sleep Medicine, 13*(4), 551–555.

K. Sexton-Radek (2013). Obstructive sleep apnea syndrome: The case of residual sleepiness. *Health, 5*(11). https://doi.org/10.4326/health.2013.5M252

K. Sutherland, O. M. Vanderveken, H. Tsuda, M. Marklund, F. Gagnadoux, C. A. Kushida, & P. A. Cistulli (2014). Oral appliance treatment for obstructive sleep apnea: An update. *Journal of Clinical Sleep Medicine, 10*(2): 215–227.

P. Strollo, M. Sooser, J. Mauren, N., Vries, J. Cornelius, R. Hanson, et al. (2014). Upper-airway Stimulation for obstructive sleep apnea. *New England Journal of Medicine, 370*(2), 139–149. https://doi.org/10.1056/NEJMOA1308659

P. A. Vanable, J. G. Aikins, L. Tadineti, B. Caruana-Montaldo, & W. B. Mendelson (2000). Sleep latency and duration estimates among sleep disorder patients: Variability as a function of sleep disorder diagnoses, sleep history and psychological characteristics. *Sleep, 23*(1), 1–9.

N. Watson, M. Badrm, G. Belenky, D. Bliwise, O. Burton, D. Buysse, et al. (2015). Joint Consensus Statement of the American Academy of Sleep Medicine and Sleep Research Society on the recommended amount of sleep for a healthy adult: Methodology and discussion. *Journal of Sleep Medicine, 11*(8), 931–952. https://doi.org/10.5665/sleep14716

K. Yaouhi, F. Bertran, P. Clochon, F. Mezenga, P. Denise, J. Foret, et al. (2009). A combined neuropsychological and brain imaging study of obstructive sleep apnea. *Journal of Sleep Research, 18*, 36–48. https://doi.org/10.1111/j.1365-2869.2008.00705.x

S. J. Yo-El, M. B. Finn, C. L. Sutphen, E. M. Herries, G. M. Jerome, J. H. Ladenson, et al. (2016). Obstructive sleep apnea decreases central nervous system-derived proteins in the cerebrospinal fluid. *Annals of Neurology, 80*(1), 154–159. https://doi.org/10.1002/ANA.24672

M. E. Zimmerman, & M. S. Aloia (2008). A review of neuroimaging in obstructive sleep apnea. *Journal of Clinical Sleep Medicine, 2*(4), 461–471.

CHAPTER 3

Restless Legs/Periodic Limb Movement Disorder

Restless legs syndrome (RLS) and periodic limb movement disorder (PLMD) are the most common movement disorders that disturb sleep. RLS produces the most profound disturbance of sleep, second only to sleep apnea. There are a myriad of health and personal factors associated with RLS. RLS was first diagnosed in the seventeenth century by a description of "extreme motor activity" and treated with opioids (opium). Some three hundred years later, further description of RLS entered the medical diagnostic world. In 1982, experimental treatments of L-Dopa and dopamine agonists led to the restoration of sleep (and discontinuance of opioid treatments).

The diagnosis of RLS includes the following components: the urge to move the legs that may or may not be accompanied by unpleasant sensory sensations (creepy, crawly, tingly sensations in legs); the urge to move the legs that may be partially or totally relieved by movement; and the need to move the legs that is not associated with another medical condition. In most RLS cases, there is a family history of the condition. RLS is experienced most commonly in the evening during presleep. A complete medical examination is necessary to rule out other causes of RLS and nerve damage (neuropathy, radical apathy), venous stasis, and claudication. The overall prevalence of RLS is approximately 10% of the general population, with the prevalence increasing with age, particularly in females over 30 years old (WebMD, 2019).

RLS tends to occur or worsen while a person is at rest. Trouble sleeping or sitting for long periods of time can be problematic. Working at one's desk; sitting in a car, bus, or train; or watching a movie in a theater can be difficult, uncomfortable, and frustrating because the urge to move the legs is overwhelming. Additionally, the frequency and severity can range from mild to unbearable, with severity worse in the evening and greatly affecting sleep onset and quality of sleep.

Abnormal central and peripheral iron regulation in RLS patients at autopsy is a commonly cited finding. More recent brain injury studies identified increased levels of dopamine, but these results are not supported. Also, suspected genetic linkage has not been found.

Quality of life is disturbed in RLS patients. The difficulty falling asleep reduces sleep time to some five hours per night. On symptom-checklist evaluations, RLS patients score higher than the general population, particularly in areas of social function and mental health. Medical evaluation entails a physical examination, iron ferritin lead levels, and vitamin-D levels. RLS is categorized in terms of intermittent, frequent, chronic, and refractory. There are medical treatment guidelines with each level. Behavioral treatments entail instruction in sleep hygiene, review of medications to determine those identified as provoking RLS (antihistamines), and sleep-schedule management and controlled napping to manage sleep quality. These interventions are done in a cognitive behavioral therapy (CBT) format.

When leg movements occur during sleep and are of a certain frequency, they are referred to as periodic limb movement disorder (PLMD). Surface electrodes measure muscle activation in each thigh as the patient sleeps to evaluate for PLMD. The number of movements per minute is categorized. Consensus viewpoints coalesce around the component of autonomic arousal. There is evidence of increased spinal motor activity in RLS and PLMD patients. PLMD most commonly occurs between the ages of 15 and 35. Transient changes in cardiovascular measures of blood pressure and heart rate co-occur with RLS and PLMD. Management of current medications and dopaminergic medications are used for treatment.

Psychological Impact of RLS/PLMD

The impact of RLS and PLMD can be seen in both the poor quality of patients' sleep, as well as the compromised daytime functioning that is secondary to excessive sleepiness from fragmented sleep. De Buisseret, Maireese, Newell, Verland, and Neu (2017) reported on the comparisons of RLS and PLMD patient responses to standard sleep measures. Greater variation in scores from the Hamilton Rating Scales of Anxiety and Depression and Fatigue Severity Scale were found for both conditions. It was concluded that the similar sleep disturbance of RLS and PLMD significantly impacted nighttime sleep and daytime functioning (De Buisseret et al., 2017). Svetel, Jovic, Pekneyovic, and Kostic (2015) identified elevations on the Hamilton Depressions and Anxiety subscales in a community-based sample of participants who self-reported RLS. Ipsiroglug et al. (2016) investigated a pediatric sample with neurodevelopmental conditions. Parental narratives describing their child's sleep were used to detect the "urge to move" feature of RLS. The plotted narratives identified "urge to move" RLS feature in 88% of the patients. In a comparison of age-matched controls and patients with RLS, Brand, Beck, Hatzinger, and Holsboer-Trachsler (2013) reported lower levels of internal locus of control, unfavorable sleep-related personality traits, low self-confidence, and higher mental arousal. A specialized questionnaire to measure personality style in sleep disordered, called the Frage Logen and Erfassung Personality Traits, determined unfavorable scores on sleep-related personality traits, such as resigned, burdened, indecisive, impaired, and concerned about sleep. Guler and Turan (2015) administered the Restless Legs Syndrome Quality of Life questionnaire to RLS patients. A reduction in the magnitude of scores on the questionnaire scales was found for the RLS patent group that did not have symptoms of insomnia compared to the group with RLS and insomnia (Guler & Turan, 2015).

RLS Impact on Medical Conditions

Woo, Lee, Hwang, and Ahn (2017) identified symptoms of RLS and PLMD in poststroke patients. Brain injury studies identified the pontine base and tegmentum lesions and unilateral RLS. Lesions in the corona radiate, and adjacent basal ganglia were associated with bilateral RLS (Woo, Lee, Hwang, & Ahn, 2017). Tekin (2015) identified impaired vagal activation of the cardiovascular system as a factor related to cardiovascular disease and RLS. Tekin (2015) suggested frame count and recording speed adjustments to measures of coronary flow to better estimate coronary flow in patients with RLS. In a case-control design, Cholley-Roulleau et al. (2017) identified RLS association to hypercholesterolemia, sleep apnea, and increased age, using a standardized questionnaire.

There is a heightened prevalence of RLS in patients with rheumatoid arthritis. In a study to discern arthritic pain from RLS, Taylor-Gjevre, Gjevre, and Nair (2014) utilized an Actigraph monitor that counts leg movements and participants' self-report measures of their rheumatic arthritis and sleep quality. The rheumatoid arthritis participants who met criteria described as RLS had a higher frequency of PLMD than those who did not have RLS (Taylor-Gjevre, Gjevre, & Nair, 2014).

Genetic studies of RLS have examined the association between Thr105I1e (rs11558538) polymorphic in the histamine-1-methyltransferase (HNMT) gene. Some RLS patients have the rs11558535TT genotype and early onset Parkinson's disease (Jimenez-Jimenez et al., 2017). RLS is also called Willis-Ekbom disease. Rinaldi et al. (2016) summarized findings from a large cohort study of RLS patients examined by physicians and sleep specialists. RLS symptoms are most commonly present in the early evening, with a smaller proportion of cases experiencing RLS within the first hour of sleep (Rinaldi et al., 2016). RLS patients with severe symptomology were found to have elevated levels of plasma apelin as compared to RLS patients with milder symptomology and age-matched controls (Korkmaz, Aksu, & Baskol, 2017).

Several medical diseases have been found to co-occur with RLS. Lin et al. (2016) reported from a fifty-study meta-analysis of the overall prevalence of chronic kidney disease and RLS at 24.2% (95% CI, 20.1–28.7). The classic migraine headache is characterized by an aura or neurological symptoms in RLS patients (Lin et al., 2016). Patients diagnosed with systemic lupus erythematosus, when experiencing anemia, have been found to be at higher risk for RLS (Kucuk et al., 2017). Liborio et al. (2013) reported higher levels of RLS in nephrotic patients with hypoalbuminemia. Additionally, reduced sleep quality was reported in these patients.

Jones and Cavanna (2013) stated that most patients with RLS have PLMD, but patients can have RLS without PLMD. Genetic variation, as explained in the previous paragraph, along with brain metabolism fluctuation, iron deficiency, coronary vascular rate abnormalities, and peripheral neuropathy (circadian alterations, dysfunctional nerve conduction) have been identified as causative factors of RLS. The earlier the onset of RLS, the more commonly a genetic dysfunction within central dopamine systems and iron metabolism is identified (Jones & Cavanna, 2013). Vitamin-D acts to increase levels of dopamine, and it metabolizes in the brain (Cakir et al., 2015).

Iron ferritin levels, laboratory measures, and a history and physical are used to diagnose RLS. An all-night sleep study is essential to the diagnoses of PLMD. The treatment is based on the diagnostic findings. In an elderly population with RLS/PLMD diagnoses, intravenous iron was a necessary treatment (Lieske, Becker, Schulz, Polidori, Kassubek, & Roehrig, 2015). Otherwise, dopamine agonist medications are used to treat RLS/PLMD (Bogan, Lee, Bachfuhrer, Jaros, Kim, & Shang, 2015; Giannaki et al., 2013).

Based on an observational cross-sectional study, Snitselaar, Smits, and Spijker (2016) identified RLS symptoms in patient participants diagnosed with attention-deficit hyperactivity disorder (ADHD)-hyperactivity-impulsivity type.

Unpleasant sensory and motor sensations in one's leg characterize RLS. Wetter and Pollmacher (1997) noted the effectiveness of dopaminergic agonists in the treatment of RLS is hypothesized to be due to irregular neuronal firings in the motor and sensory.

The literature states many "triggers" may aggravate RLS symptomatology. For example, common medicines, both prescription and nonprescription, can aggravate RLS/PLMD (Rottach et al., 2008; WebMD, 2019):

Antidepressants
 8–9% overall occurrence (the worst being mirtazapine)
Anti-nausea medication (e.g., Zofran)
Beta blockers (e.g., angiotensin-converting enzyme [ACE] inhibitors)
Antidopaminergic medications (e.g., metoclopramide, prochlorperazine)
Over-the-counter sleep aids and cold remedies (e.g., diphenhydramine,
 ephedrine, and pseudoephedrine)

Additional triggers include but are not limited to being still; sleep deprivation; extreme temperatures (hot and humid weather, cold weather); alcohol, sugar, and caffeine intake (including chocolate); smoking; and stress. If ingestion of sugar, caffeine, and alcohol aggravates RLS symptoms, removing these types of foods from one's diet may be helpful. For those individuals who smoke, quitting smoking may be of great benefit.

Treatment

Many of the triggers for RLS also affect PLMD. The same is true for the medications that treat RLS—they also treat PLMD. Medications often used to treat RLS symptoms are dopaminergic drugs. This classification of drugs interacts with dopamine in the brain and treats the nerve pain associated with RLS. For example, Mirapex, Requip, and Neupro are Food and Drug Administration (FDA)-approved dopaminergic drugs that treat moderate to severe RLS (WebMD, 2019). Another class of drugs, anticonvulsants, can also produce some relief. Commonly prescribed anticonvulsant medications are Tegretol, Neurontin, and

Lyrica. Narcotic pain relievers can also be prescribed; long-term use of this class of medications must be carefully watched to avoid addiction or physical dependence. While benzodiazepines may help with sleep onset and assist with relaxation, the side effect can include daytime sleepiness. There are also holistic approaches to RLS treatment, such as nutritional supplements (e.g., magnesium) and acupuncture. Holistic approaches have been scrutinized for their efficacy in relieving RLS symptoms. In addition to medications to treat RLS, additional treatments may be helpful to RLS patients. Due to the nocturnal frequency of PLMD (it occurs during sleep), these may not be helpful for PLMD patients.

Leg massages often help relieve the RLS symptoms. The massages can be done by a professional massage therapist, the person afflicted with RLS, or another person. There are leg massage devices that also offer relief. Additionally, hot baths are also helpful in alleviating the RLS symptomatology. Some RLS patients add aromatic oils to the hot baths, and those patients with access to whirlpool-style bathtubs often find this helpful, if not relaxing. RLS patients are cautioned to not set the temperature so hot that they are scalded by the hot water.

Some patients have reported finding relief from heating pads or ice packs. There are a variety of heating pads and ice packs that are designed to fit the contour of the leg. Individual differences will dictate whether heat or cold is helpful. Some patients report altering between hot and cold is beneficial in the relief of RLS symptomatology.

Exercise may help achieve relief from RLS symptomatology. Patients have reported that including exercise in their daily schedules, especially taking a walk prior to bedtime, has eased symptoms. Stretching has also been found helpful if done close to bedtime. If one chooses to exercise early in the day, it may aggravate RLS.

Stress has been shown to be a trigger for RLS; however, engaging in stress relief has been shown to be efficacious. Behaviors or activities that reduce anxiety, tension, and stress are beneficial. For example, engaging in meditation, guided imagery, deep breathing, and yoga can promote relaxation and decrease stress/anxiety.

Effects and Costs

At Work

RLS patients have higher levels of work absenteeism, presenteeism, and overall productivity loss (*National Health and Wellness Survey*, 2012).

In Personal Lives

RLS patients have significantly lower health-related quality of life. Trying to "quiet" the symptoms of RLS affects their ability to engage in all aspects of life. Medications may not relieve the RLS symptoms and the discomfort can vary from mild to extreme. RLS patients also experience a greater economic and humanistic burden than non-RLS patients (*National Health and Wellness Survey*, 2012). For instance, RLS patients experience higher rates of absenteeism from employment, disengagement from social activities, higher health provider visits and hospitalization than non-RLS patients resulting in greater economic burdens.

Case Study: RLS without PLMD

Deedee is a 33-year-old female married graduate student who was self-referred for uncomfortable, tingly/prickly leg sensations, and a feeling of "soda pop running down her legs and in her veins." She was accompanied by her husband. He stated that she occasionally kicked her legs at night. Deedee denied kicking her legs during sleep. She stated that she often cannot get comfortable due to the unpleasant leg sensations, and these often kept her awake at night. She stated that movement relieved her sensations; however, she was a graduate student and attended classes in the evening and stated that the urge to move her legs in class was often disruptive. She described her classroom size as small, with approximately seven students sitting in conference-room-style seating. She had to get up and pace the room, and she noticed that the students and teacher often get frustrated because she cannot stay still. It is for this reason that she presented to the sleep clinic.

Deedee is of normal body habitus. She had a neck circumference of 13 inches and was 5 foot, 4 inches tall and weighed 123 pounds. Her husband and she denied snoring or periods when she stopped breathing during the night, acting out dreams, sleep paralysis (waking up unable to move), experiencing hallucinations, sleep walking, or sleep eating. She denied a significant medical history and was not taking any prescription or over-the-counter medications. She denied a history of depression or anxiety.

She stated that if her leg "issues" were present, she had a difficult time falling asleep and did not wake up feeling refreshed. She often had difficulty concentrating during the day, especially at school and when trying to complete her homework assignments. On days and nights when she was symptom free, she fell asleep without issue and woke up feeling refreshed. She denied waking up to use the restroom at night.

When interviewed regarding her dietary intake, she admitted to smoking (three to five cigarettes per day), drinking four or five cans of caffeinated soda per day, eating chocolate (three to five pieces per day), and generally ordering fast food because she did not have time to cook food and often snacked on cake and candy. Deedee admitted to drinking alcohol on the weekend when she went out with her friends from graduate school (two or three beers per night). She denied engaging in physical activity or exercise.

Deedee was scheduled for an overnight sleep study called a polysomnogram (PSG) to determine if she had PLMD. Results of the PSG revealed significant RLS symptoms that interfered with sleep onset, but she did not have PLMD. She spent more time in stage 1 and 2 sleep than NREM and REM stages, and there was no evidence of another sleep disorder, such as OSA.

When Deedee returned for her PSG results, she was not surprised that she had RLS and was "happy" that she did not have PLMD. Most of the visit focused on RLS education, including medications and foods or circumstances that can trigger or aggravate RLS. She was unwilling to avoid caffeine, sugar, alcohol, or smoking. She described that smoking, drinking socially on the weekends, and eating her cakes and candies were relaxing to her. She also stated that she would not give up drinking soda but would consider switching to decaffeinated soda. She agreed that graduate school was stressful but until she finished her PhD, she would have to "put up with the stress." Relaxation strategies were discussed, and she was receptive to try listening to relaxation CDs and looking into evening yoga or stretching classes.

She was prescribed a dopaminergic medication and was educated about this class of medications. Deedee stated that she was eager to try the medication because she was open to anything that would offer relief. The session focused on nonmedical strategies to help lessen RLS symptoms. Her husband was very willing to provide leg massages, and she stated that she enjoyed taking hot baths but often did not have time to do so; she would be willing to add this to her nightly routine.

Deedee returned for a one-month follow-up and stated that the medication provided 50% relief, and she was grateful. The sleep clinician increased her RLS medication to see if a change in dosage caused further relief. She stated that the nightly leg massages had been great and were mentally and physically beneficial. She noticed that she went to bed feeling more relaxed. On the nights that she had leg massages, she did not take a hot bath. The hot baths had been helpful, and she would continue having them. Last, she stated that she was still not willing to avoid the sugars, alcohol, and caffeinated food and drinks or give up smoking at the present time, even though she was aware of the association with triggering RLS. She declined trying to experiment with avoiding these trigger foods and drinks for two days to see if she felt a difference.

She returned two weeks later to see if the change in medication was effective. Deedee stated that she felt an additional 20–25% improvement, and she was less disruptive in class because the urge to move her legs was not as severe as it was. She stated that she and her husband joined an RLS support group, and she was learning that her eating, drinking, and smoking behaviors were most likely aggravating her RLS symptoms. Her husband stated that she was now drinking caffeine-free soda and reduced her smoking to one or two cigarettes per day. She was not willing to make any additional changes but was highly praised for her behavior changes.

Deedee moved out of state six months after her initial appointment and was lost to follow-up. At her last appointment, she stated that the RLS severity was downgraded from severe to mild-to-moderate symptoms. She attributed the reduction of RLS symptomatology and severity to medication management. Even though she was able to reduce her smoking intake and change to drinking caffeine-free soda, she was not willing to make any further changes in eating sugary foods and limiting alcohol. She was still eating chocolate daily as of her last visit. The clinician postulates about how much improvement Deedee would have received in both the severity and frequency of RLS symptoms if she had made additional changes to her trigger foods and behaviors.

Case Study: PLMD and RLS Diagnoses

Ron is a 63-year-old widowed male who presented with daytime sleepiness and pain in his legs (feeling of spiders walking on his legs) and reported waking himself up at night when his legs twitch or kick. He often woke up not feeling refreshed. He was accompanied by his daughter, who stated that her father often looked tired and had been found walking around his neighborhood at night because he often needed to move his legs to alleviate the discomfort that he felt. She stated that he was found walking one mile from his home by a police officer who drove him home for fear that his safety might be threatened by walking in the dark and being alone.

Ron reported that he was a retired NASA engineer who worked on "top-secret space equipment." He was 5 foot, 10 inches tall and had a slender body habitus. He had a fifteen-inch neck circumference. He stated that he exercised with free weights and did cardio training at his home three to five days per week. He emphasized the importance of eating healthy because he had a family history of cardiac disease. His only significant medical history was arthritis, which did not limit his daily functioning. Blood testing revealed no abnormalities or issues of clinical significance.

He denied experiencing snoring, acting out his dreams, periods when he stopped breathing, taking daily naps, hallucinations, or sleep paralysis. If he felt sleepy during the day, he avoided napping and started to exercise. His bedtime varied depending on if his "legs are being problematic." He went to bed anytime between 8:00 and 11:30 p.m. He denied drinking alcohol, smoking, or having caffeine drinks or foods with caffeine after 4:00 p.m. Ron stated that he would have a cup of coffee first thing upon arising (approximately 7:00 a.m.) and may have a slice of cake with his coffee. He generally refrained from sweet foods because he did not want to gain weight and denied eating chocolate.

Ron was scheduled for an overnight PSG test. The results revealed that he had both RLS and moderate PLMD, which affected both sleep onset and sleep maintenance. Treatment would focus on medication management and behavioral changes.

Ron and his daughter presented for his follow-up PSG appointment. The clinician revealed the results of his PSG and focused on education regarding medications in management of both RLS and PLMD. The session also focused on which medications, foods, and behaviors can trigger leg movements and activities to engage in to help alleviate leg movement complaints.

Ron was prescribed dopaminergic medication to assist with relief of both RLS and nocturnal kicking leg movements associated with PLMD. Ron was already educated on the dopaminergic drugs and asked appropriate questions, such as how long he would need to be on the medication and what side effects he might experience. He was informed that management of both RLS and PLMD is lifelong. While medication will not "cure" the disease, it can very likely produce a major reduction in symptoms, allowing for restful, undisturbed sleep and an increase in quality of life.

The clinician focused on discussing triggers for RLS and PLMD. Ron stated that he did not stay up late at night, and while he had an active social life, he tried to keep a scheduled bedtime and wake routine. He would try to move his exercise routine to late afternoon or early evening. His daughter stated that her father was a perfectionist, which can add to stress if he did not accomplish something the way he felt it should be done. For instance, he was working with his oldest grandchild, who wanted his help in making a go-cart. He was able to perfect the dynamics of the go-cart design, but building the go-cart was difficult because of his arthritic joints, and the overall completion of the go-cart was not to his "satisfaction." Ron was amenable to trying deep breathing or meditation exercises. He stated that he was going to sign up at the YMCA to take tai chi classes to help with his joint mobility and with decreasing stress, as well as the overall health benefits.

When discussing nonmedication treatments, his daughter stated that she purchased a leg massage device—a chair that he sat in and the legs were wrapped in a massage device that provided warmth during the massage function. He also stated that he would begin to use his whirlpool bath again at night because he enjoyed the benefits of the hot water.

A follow-up appointment was scheduled for two weeks later, and Ron stated that he was sleeping throughout the night and waking up feeling alert. His RLS had decreased significantly, and the leg massage equipment and taking hot baths in his whirlpool bath were both very beneficial. He definitely felt more relaxed, and he denied having to walk the neighborhood before bedtime. Last, he was enjoying his tai chi classes and felt that in addition to the medication management, he was able to do things to help his leg movement issues, which made him feel empowered.

Follow-up appointments revealed that he continued to sleep well and was engaging in his nonmedication activities. At his last appointment, he stated that he was surprised "an old man like him" could still make powerful changes in his life that could affect overall wellness. He took his medication daily and enjoyed what he described as a "bougie" lifestyle of spa-like massage equipment and hot baths.

Case Study
Rene was a 49-year-old married female employed as a clinical researcher. Her husband accompanied her to the visit and stated that she often woke him up during sleep because she kicked during her sleep. She stated that she awakened at night often due to her leg movements and woke up feeling "slightly" refreshed. She denied taking naps during the day because she was busy at work, but stated that she did feel tired at times during the day.

She was 5 foot, 7 inches tall and weighs 158 pounds. Her neck circumference was 13 inches. She stated that she ran five miles in the morning before going to work and denied drinking alcohol, smoking, or eating sugary foods. She did have one to three cups of coffee, but her last cup of coffee was at 1:00 p.m. She denied having difficulty falling asleep or staying asleep or early morning awakenings, unpleasant leg sensations, snoring, periods when she stopped breathing during sleep, hallucinations, or sleep paralysis. Her husband agreed with the denial of these symptoms.

Her medical history was significant for anxiety, which was controlled by taking Lexapro 10 mg. Blood testing revealed no deficiencies or abnormalities. She stated that she had three children, aged 5, 9, and 12. She often worked long hours developing drugs for a large biotech company. While she stated that she enjoys her work, it was stressful, and her manager tended to micromanage all his employees, which created an unpleasant working environment. She described herself as a "type-A personality" and wanted to ensure everything was done well.

She and her husband were currently in marriage counseling because she suffered a miscarriage six months into her pregnancy, and they were finding it difficult to cope with the loss. She stated that she and her husband were doing well, but they decided not to have any additional children.

Based on Rene's and her husband's reports of leg movements at night, she was scheduled for a PSG. Results revealed that she had a periodic leg movement index of 45, which is classified as moderate periodic leg movements. Light snoring not associated with arousal was noted, but it did not disturb sleep, and Rene's husband denied that she snores. All other sleep events were within normal limits.

Rene and her husband presented for a follow-up appointment after her PSG. Results were provided to her, and she was not surprised by the diagnosis. She was surprised at the snoring and stated that she felt congested during the sleep study, which may have impacted the results.

Medication management was discussed, and Rene was willing to start taking a prescribed dopaminergic medication. Treatment compliance was discussed, as well as the side effects of treatment. Rene was aware of the side effects of the dopaminergic medications. Prior to her appointment, she had researched treatment regimens for PLMD. She asked if she would have to take the medication long-term, and she was educated that if she stopped taking the medication, there was a high probability that the leg movement symptoms would return.

A follow-up appointment was scheduled for one month after her appointment because Rene and her family were taking a three-week vacation. After her vacation, she returned for her follow-up appointment and stated that she felt a "vast" improvement. Her husband stated that she had not been kicking him during her sleep so they were both sleeping through the night. Overall, she felt really well and had more energy and focus during the day. She was asked to return in one month.

She presented alone without her husband for the follow-up visit. She continued to feel great and sleep well. Her husband continued to deny being awoken due to her "kicking him." She continued to report feeling stress at work and stated that she was scheduling an appointment with a cognitive behavioral therapist to assist with stress reduction. She also stated that she and her husband were no longer in marital therapy and that things continued to be good between them.

Six months after the results of her polysomnogram, she called the clinic stating that her husband was noting that she was starting to kick during her sleep, but it was mild in frequency. Her neurologist made a medication change (increased her medication), and she was asked to return to the clinic in two weeks.

She and her husband returned to the clinic in two weeks, and her husband stated that she was no longer kicking in her sleep. Rene stated that she continued to feel well and, since the medication change, had more energy. She started therapy and had been working with her psychologist on addressing work-associated stress. She was also in the process of trying to find a new job.

Six months later, Rene stated that her manager was fired, and she was promoted to be the new manager. She stated that her level of stress had greatly declined; she was enjoying work. Her recent annual review was very positive, and overall, she rated her quality of life as excellent, especially that she no longer had to "deal with" PLMD affecting her life.

Case Study

Wilma was a 24-year-old single, pregnant female who was a full-time college student. She presented to the sleep clinic because of complaints of "weird" sensations in her legs (e.g., feeling tingling and burning, as well as charley horse sensations) that occur mostly in the late afternoon and evenings. She stated that the symptoms began three months into her pregnancy, and she was currently eight months pregnant. She denied having leg movements during her sleep but did not have a bed partner who could confirm or deny leg movements.

She was 5 foot, 1 inch and weighed 133 pounds. Her neck circumference was 15 inches. She denied snoring, periods when she stopped breathing, sleep paralysis, and hallucinations. She did endorse feeling sleepy during the day and did not wake feeling refreshed. Her Epworth sleepiness scale revealed that she was mildly sleepy during the day. She denied falling asleep while working, studying, and driving, but would fall asleep if she was watching evening television.

She stated that moving her legs helped alleviate the discomfort. She also noticed that walking prior to going to bed helped as well. She denies smoking, drinking alcohol (only when not pregnant and on a social basis), and use of recreational drugs. Wilma stated that she often bought pies and pastries to eat because they are not expensive, and would have chocolate occasionally. She drank caffeinated beverages such as coffee, iced tea, and energy drinks. She stated that her medical history is not significant for any diseases or disorders and she was not currently taking any medications except prenatal vitamins. Results of her blood testing were within limits.

Because she was eight months pregnant, she would return to the clinic after the birth of her baby to see if her leg complaints were resolved. RLS can occur with pregnancy, and since she did not have a bed partner to confirm if there might be additional concerns with sleep, the polysomnogram (PSG) would be scheduled at a later date. During the visit, education regarding "trigger" foods, medications, and behaviors was discussed. Wilma was not aware that drinking caffeine could aggravate her leg sensations. She stated that she would try to decrease if not give up drinking caffeinated beverages.

Wilma returned to the clinic three months after the birth of her daughter and stated that leg complaints had gotten about 40% better. She reunited with the father of her daughter, and he stated that she not only snored loudly, but she also kicked him during the night. Her Epworth Sleep Score did not change; she remained in the mildly sleepy category. She continued to deny automobile accidents and falling asleep while studying or working.

She was scheduled for an overnight PSG. Results revealed that she had loud snoring and mild apneic events associated with obstructive sleep apnea. These periods of breathing cessation tended to occur more while sleeping on her back. Her snoring was not associated with arousals. She had mild kicking movements that occurred when she was having an apneic episode.

She and her boyfriend returned for discussion of her PSG results. She was surprised by her results. Treatments for OSA were discussed. She stated that she did not want to be prescribed CPAP or an oral appliance or have a surgical procedure in her mouth, but she was open to weight reduction and learning position therapy to avoid sleeping on her back.

She stated that while she lost most of her pregnancy weight, she still wanted to reduce her weight by 20 pounds, which she felt would improve her sleep quality. She asked for a nutritionist referral which was provided. Wilma also stated that since she was taking a year off from school, she would start to walk with her baby in a stroller as a weight-reduction strategy. She stated that she would give up her energy drinks because they have calories and sugar in them but would continue to have her morning coffee. She also stated that her leg sensations (burning, tingling sensations) were no longer present.

She called the sleep clinic 3 months after her appointment and stated that she had lost 10 pounds and was feeling better and healthier. Her boyfriend stated that she was not snoring as loudly or as much, and he did not notice any periods where she stopped breathing. He also stated that Wilma was not kicking him in her sleep.

Five months after her initial PSG results appointment, she stated that she had lost a total of 30 pounds and was feeling great and energized. She stated that losing the extra weight through changes in her diet and adding physical exercise had been an excellent strategy. Her boyfriend stated that she no longer snored and had not kicked him during the night for almost four months. They were both sleeping well, and she reported waking up feeling refreshed. Her mother had been staying with her and had been helping with nighttime care of her child. This support has allowed her to sleep, and the predominant reason that she was waking up feeling refreshed was that she did not have to wake up and attend to her child.

She stated that since her mother was helping with caring for her daughter, she was applying for full-time employment because she could use the extra money before resuming her school attendance. She stated that while changing her eating behaviors and eating choices had been difficult initially, it became second nature to her in a short time. Adding the exercise strategy was also initially difficult because she was "out of shape," but she now looks forward to exercising.

In this case, Wilma's leg movements were associated with OSA, and there was no need for medication; however, if her leg movements were to continue to occur outside of the apneic events and despite OSA treatment, that would necessitate medication management for treatment of PLMD. Additionally, since Wilma had mild OSA, weight reduction strategies were able to eliminate OSA.

References

R. K. Bogan, D. O. Lee, M. J. Bunfuhrer, M. J. Jaros, R. Kim, & G Shang (2015). Treatment response to sleep, pain, and mood disturbance and their correlates with sleep disturbance in adult patients with moderate-to-severe primary restless legs syndrome: Pooled analysis from 3 trials of gabapentin enacarbil. *Annals of Medicine, 47*, 269–277.

S. Brand, J Beck, M. Hatzinger, & E. Holsboer-Trachsler (2013). Patient suffering from restless legs syndrome have low internal locus of control and poor psychological functioning compared to health controls. *Neurospychobiology, 68*, 51–58.

T. Cakir, G. Dogan, V. Subasi, M. B. Filiz, N. Ulker, S. K. Dogan, & N. Toraman (2015). An evaluation of sleep quality and the prevalence of restless leg syndrome in Vitamin D deficiency. *ACTA Neurology Belgium, 115*, 623–627.

M. Cholley-Roulleau, S. Chenini, S. Bezlat, L. Guirad, I. Jaussent, & Y. Dauvilliers (2017). Restless legs syndrome and cardiovascular diseases: A case-control study. *PLoS One*. http://doi:org/10.1371/journal.pone.0176552

T. Dargin, E. A. Witt, & J. Fishman (2015). The humanistic and economic burden of restless legs syndrome. *PLoS One*. https://doi.org/10.1371/journal.pone.O140632

F. X. De Buisseret, O. Mairess, J. Newell, P. Verbanck, & D. Neu (2017). While isolated periodic limb movement disorder significantly impacts sleep depth and efficiency, co-morbid restless leg syndrome mainly exacerbates perceived sleep quality. *European Neurology, 77*, 272–280.

P. Elshoff, W. Cawello, J. O. Andreas, F. X. Mathy, & M. Braun (2015). An update on pharmacological, pharmacokinetic properties and drug-drug interaction of Rotigotine transdermal system in Parkinson's disease and restless legs syndrome. *Drugs, 75*, 487–501.

C. D. Giannaki, G. K. Sakkas, C. Karazafen, G. M. Hadjigeorgiou, E. Laudas, T. Kyriakidis, et al. (2013). Effects of exercise training and dopamine agonist in patients with uremic restless legs syndrome: A six-month randomized, partially double-blind, placebo-controlled comparative study. *Biomedical Central Nephrology, 14*, 194. https://doi.org/1471-2369/14/194

S. Guller, & F. N. Turan (2015). Turkish version of Johns Hopkins Restless Legs Syndrome Quality of Life Questionnaire (RLS-QOL): Validity and Reliability Study. *Quality of Life Research, 24*, 2789–2794.

S. J. Hoogwaut, M. V. Paananen, A. J. Smith, D. J. Beales, P. B. O'Sullivan, L. M. Straker, et al. (2015). Musculoskeletal pain is associated with restless legs syndrome in young adults. *BioMedCentral Musculoskeletal Disorders*. https://doi.org/10.1186/s/2891-015-0765-1

O. S. Ipsiroglug, N. Beyzael, M. Berger, A. L. Wagner, S. Dhalla, J. Garden, & S. Stockler (2016). Emplotted narratives and structured behavioral observation supporting the diagnoses of Willis-Ekbom Disease/Restless Leg Syndrome in children with neurodevelopmental conditions. *Neuroscience & Therapeutics, 22,* 894–905.

F. J. Jimenez-Jimenez, E. G. Martin, H. Alonso-Navarro, C. Martinex, M. Zurdo, L. Turapin-Fendl, et al. (2017). Thr105IIe (RS11558538) polymorphism in the histamine-l-methyl-transferase (HNMT) gene and risk for restless legs syndrome. *Journal of Neuro Transmission, 124,* 285–291. https://doi.org/10.1007/s00702-016-1645-z

R. Jones, & A. Cavanna (2013). The neurobiology and treatment of restless legs syndrome. *Behavioral Neurology, 26,* 283–292.

F. Kocabicak, M. Terzi, K. Akpinar, K. Paksay, I. Cebeci, & O. Lyigan (2014). Restless leg syndrome and sleep quality in lumbar radiculopathy patients. *Behavioral Neurology,* Article ID 245358, https://doi.org/10.1144/2014/245358

A. L. Komaroff (2013). *Ask the doctor restless leg treatment.* Retrieved May 30, 2021, from https://www.health.harvard.edu/diseases-and-conditions/restless-leg-treatments

S. Korkmaz, M. Aksu, & G. Baskol (2017). Plasma apelin level in patients with restless legs syndrome and its association with periodic leg movements. *Sleep Breath, 21,* 19–24. https://doi.org/10.107/s11325-016-1355-7

A. Kucuk, A. Uslu, R. Yilmaz, E. Salbas, Y. Solar, & R. Tunc (2017). Relationship between prevalence and severity of restless legs syndrome and anemia in patients with systemic lupus erythematosus. *International Journal of Rheumatic Diseases, 20,* 469–473.

A. B. Liborio, J. P. Santos, N. R. Minote, A. Doyenes, L. A. Faria, & V. M. deBruin (2013). Restless legs syndrome and quality of sleep in patients with glomerulopathy. *Biomedical Central Nephrology, 14,* 113.

B. Lieske, I. Becker, R. J. Schulz, M. C. Polidori, J. Kassubek & G. Roehrig (2016). Intravenous iron administration in restless legs syndrome: An observational study. *Journal of Gerontology and Geriatrics, 49,* 626–631.

G. Y. Lin, J. T. Lee, M. S. Lee, C. C. Lin, C. K. Tsai, D. H. Ting, & F. C Yang (2016). Prevalence of restless legs syndrome in migraine patients with and without aura: A cross-sectional, case-controlled study. *The Journal of Headache and Pain, 17,* 97. https://doi.org/10.18618/s10194-016-0691-0

Z. Lin, C. Zhao, Q. Luo, X. Xia, X. Yu, & F. Huang (2016). Prevalence of restless leg syndrome in chronic kidney disease: A systematic review and meta-analysis of observational studies. *Renal Failure, 38*(9), 1335–1346.

S. Mackie, & J. W. Winkelman (2015). Long term treatment of restless legs syndrome (RLS): An approach to management of worsening symptoms, loss of efficacy and augmentation. *CNS Drugs, 29,* 351–357.

National Health and Wellness Survey. 2012. Kantar Group and Affiliates, London. www.kantar.com

A. Q. Rana, H. R. Qurshi, L. Rahman, A. Jesudasan, K. K. Hafez, & M. A. Rana (2015). Association of restless leg syndrome, pain, and mood disorders in Parkinson's disease. *International Journal of Neuroscience, 162*(2), 111–120.

F. Rinaldi, A. Galbiata, S. Marelli, M. Cusmai, A. Gasper, A. Oldani, et al. (2016). Defining the phenotype of restless legs syndrome/Willis–Ekbom disease (RLS/WED): A clinical and polysomnographic study. *Journal of Neurology, 263,* 396–402. https://doi.org/10.1007/s00415-015-7994-y

K. G. Rottach, B. M. Schaner, M. H. Kirch, A. Z. Zivotofsky, L. M. Teufel, T. Gallwitz, & T. Messer (2008). Restless legs syndrome as side effect of second generation antidepressants. *Journal of Psychiatric Research, 43*(1), 70–75.

M. A. Snitselaar, M. G. Smits, & J. Spijker (2016). Prevalence of restless legs syndrome in adult ADHD and its subtypes. *Behavioral Sleep Medicine, 14,* 480–488.

M. V. Svetel, J. Jovic, T. D. Pegnezovic, & V. Kostic (2015). Quality of Life in patients with primary restless legs syndrome. Community-based study. *Neurological Science, 36,* 1345–1351.

R. Taylor-Gjevre, J. D. Gjevre, & B. U. Nair (2014). Increased nocturnal periodic limb movements in rheumatoid arthritis patients meeting questionnaire diagnostic criteria for restless leg syndrome. *BioMedCentral Musculoskeletal Disorders, 15,* 378. https://doi.org/10.1186/1471-2474-15-378

G. Tekin (2015). Restless leg syndrome and slow coronary flow. Is it inflammation or autonomic nervous system? *Anatolian Journal Cardiology, 15:* 509–514.

WebMD (2019). *Restless legs syndrome (RLS)*. Retrieved December 31, 2019, from https://www.webmd.com/brain/restless-legs-syndrome/restless-legs-syndrome-rls#1

T. C. Wetter, & T. Pollmächer (1997). Restless legs and periodic leg movements in sleep syndromes. *Journal of Neurology, 244* (Suppl. 1), S37–S45.

H. G. Woo, D. Lee, K. J. Hwang, & T. B. Ahn (2017). Post stroke restless les syndrome and periodic limb movement in sleep. *ACTA Neurological Scandinavia, 135*, 204–210. https://doi.org/10.1111

S. Yilmaz, B. Cigdem, S. F. Gokce, S. C. Dogan, & H. Balaban (2017). Severity and frequency of restless legs syndrome in patients with familial Mediterranean fever. *Journal of International Medical Research, 43*(4), 1340–1346. https://doi.org/10.1177/03000605/7704789

CHAPTER 4

Pain and Sleep

Everyone has experienced physical pain, and the intensity of the pain can vary. For some individuals, pain can vary from minimal to intense pain, but recovery tends to be quicker than for more serious conditions (e.g., bone or muscle bruise, foot blister, etc.). For less serious pain conditions, healing can be more rapid, and medical intervention is not generally required. However, for those instances where the pain can be intense, such as in a fractured ankle, the acute pain can significantly impact a patient's life, and a longer period for healing may be required. For those instances when chronic pain occurs (arthritis, bone cancer, degenerative diseases, migraines), treatment to relieve the pain may be more difficult, and treatment regimens can be more complex.

Many bodily systems are affected by pain, and one of the effects is that pain interferes with both quality and quantity of sleep. For example, if someone breaks a bone, the first night of trying to fall asleep and maintain sleep can be challenging. The throbbing and pain associated with movement both affect a person's comfort level. Try sleeping through a migraine. Yes, medication can assist with the pain and discomfort, but even some of the strongest medicines will not control pain effectively to achieve a solid night of consolidated, refreshing sleep. This chapter will focus on the difference between acute pain and chronic pain, treatment of pain, and its relationship to sleep.

In cases of chronic pain, the pain is the main focus in a patient's life. Living with chronic pain can significantly lower quality of life and can lead to the cancelling of social events (such as dinner at a friend or family's home), preventing a patient from participating in all levels of functioning.

In these cases, pain becomes a recurrent and sometimes constant problem that assumes a central role in a patient's daily lives. Treatments for both acute and chronic pain are available; however, some patients avoid pain medications and want to "push through the pain." It is important to note that treatment for pain does not have to only involve taking a prescribed medication. Physical therapy is often the number-one choice for pain management, depending on the cause of the pain, patient's pain tolerance level, and whether the pain is acute or chronic. If one is experiencing pain (acute or chronic), trying to sleep can be difficult and fragmented and can lead to not feeling refreshed upon waking.

From a historical perspective, pain has been a major focus of medical complaints and treatment plans. The problem is a notable one given that chronic, disabling pain affects over 50 million people in the United States (the number of Americans who suffer from pain [Association for Behavioral and Cognitive Therapies (ACBT), 2020; Center for Disease Control (CDC), 2018]). The 2015 Sleep in America™ Poll finds that 21% of Americans experience chronic pain and 36% have had acute pain in the past week (Sleepfoundation, 2020). Those combine to indicate that the majority of the nation's adult population, 57%, experience pain, leaving 43% who report being pain free. Chronic, disabling pain is estimated to affect over 50 million people in the United States alone (ACBT, 2020; Sleepfoundation, 2020). The costs, both monetary and personal, are substantial. For example, the leading cause of disability in working-age people is due to musculoskeletal disorder (James et al., 2018). The common cold is the second reason for absenteeism. Unfortunately, pain is a major cause for the loss of 700 million workdays and the payment of $65 billion in medical expenses annually (ACBT, 2020). The emotional, physical, and financial cost of individual suffering and the disruption of family life and career are extensive and significant.

The understanding of "pain" has undergone many dimensional concepts, ranging from viewing pain as nothing more than a physiological alarm system to warn that damage is occurring to the body to the more current concept that pain is a multifactorial concept that can occur as either acute or chronic pain. Removing pain from the body is more complicated than just curing the injury or illness. However, this concept has not been widely accepted. Physicians witnessed that patients were still complaining long after the "healing" occurred, and in some instances, pain still occurred in patients when there was no physical root cause for the pain (ACBT, 2020). What was even more puzzling to physicians was that some patients with serious physical disorders reported very mild pain and minimum disruption of daily activities.

Sadly, those patients where there was no physical explanation for the cause of their pain were labeled as mentally ill, attention seekers, and so on. Those individuals who had "little" complaints but had a physical cause for their pain were perceived as "strong" (ACBT, 2020). The ACBT authors further explained that patients were fearful of being labeled "crazy" or "weak," so they may have been reluctant to complain if there was no physical reason for the pain. Those patients with chronic pain may have been ignored by their treating physicians with the rationale that if there was no cause or explanation, how could the condition be treated? Other physicians may have provided a treatment plan that focused on relieving the chronic pain by providing "long-term" pain medication and physical and psychological therapies. This plan was the preferable one, but most physicians did not provide a treatment plan focusing on the physical and psychological rehabilitation.

ACBT (2020) provides a review of the health care community perception in 1960, where the focus for the view of chronic pain and the treatment approaches was a major change. Clinicians started to incorporate behavioral and rehabilitation approaches because chronic pain was now viewed as a multifactorial concept that resulted from the interaction between physical and emotional/psychological factors. This multifactorial approach to understanding the pain experience also focused on how behaviors and disability accompany chronic pain. This new approach to understanding pain and pain treatment separated acute pain from chronic pain.

The International Association for the Study of Pain defines pain as "an unpleasant sensory and emotional experience associated with actual or potential damage or described in terms of such damage" (Hill, 2017). Pain is traditionally dichotomized into acute and chronic. Acute pain, an indicator of potential tissue damage, may be viewed as an adaptive alarm to the physical body that warrants attention to the cause of the pain and acts as a motivator to prevent damage to the body and to avoid similar situations. For instance, from an evolutionary perspective, if there is a plant that yields fruit but obtaining the fruit will result in ant bites all over your arm, you will be less likely to put your arm in the center of the plant to avoid the stinging pain of the ant bite. Treatment for acute pain is generally treated biomedically (Lumley et al., 2011).

Chronic, or persistent, pain is defined as lasting at least three months and is more complicated than acute pain (Lumley et al., 2011). These authors further stated that pain can be maintained from learning via neurobiological, psychological, and social changes. The adaptive alarm that is associated with acute pain loses some of its efficiency because pain is no longer a reliable indicator of tissue damage, and behavioral changes to reduce pain may be maladaptive or dysfunctional (Lumley et al., 2011; Nesse & Ellsworth, 2009). Furthermore, chronic pain patients are more likely to utilize pain clinics or counseling. Treating chronic pain to resolve sleep issues can be difficult because pain may not be the only driving factor of sleep disturbance.

Treatment of Chronic Pain

Chronic pain is not a simple concept to understand because there are many factors affecting the cause and duration of the pain. For instance, there are many biological, psychological, emotional, physical, and stress factors that can exacerbate the cycle of pain. If someone has limitations due to chronic pain, depression can occur. Limiting work, physical, social, and other interactions negatively impact one's mood. Depression, sleep, and pain are related to each other. Treatment of pain varies from patient to patient according to how long, how severe, and how debilitating it is (Multiple Chronic Conditions Resource Center, 2020).

Before any treatment plan can be recommended, chronic pain must be assessed. A thorough intake of a patient's medical history must be taken, including a review of all comorbid illnesses and current medications, when the injury or pain began, pain location and intensity, potential causes of pain, what makes it better or worse, discussion of patient's beliefs about pain and coping skills, previous and current treatments, and functional impairment. Assessments of pain, sleep, and quality of life can be administered to the patient. Unless the sleep impairment is due to a primary sleep disorder (e.g., pain associated with restless leg syndrome), an overnight polysomnogram will not be conducted. Review of the clinical intake findings and assessments will aid in providing an efficacious treatment plan, which may include medication management, rehabilitation to aid in muscle and movement recovery, cognitive behavioral therapy, psychotherapy, sleep hygiene education, acupuncture, relaxation therapy, guided imagery, and so on.

Approaches that can minimize pain or assist in patient recovery include, but not limited to, cognitive, biological, behavioral, and surgical treatments to address the emotional, psychological, functional, and physical aspects of pain.

1. Cognitive Behavioral Therapy (CBT). Addresses the emotional-physical and behavioral aspects of pain. CBT follows a structured approach that focuses on the interactions and relationships

between cognitions (thoughts), emotions, and behaviors. CBT treatments can be efficacious applied as a single technique or in a combined pain management program. Evidence suggests that CBT for chronic pain improves functioning and quality of life for a variety of chronic pain conditions (Hoffman, Papas, Chatkoff, & Kerns, 2007; Murphy et al., 2020; Turner, Mancl, & Aaron, 2006). CBT for chronic pain is an approach that encourages clients to adopt an active, problem-solving approach to cope with the many challenges associated with chronic pain (Burns et al., 2014). The overarching goal of CBT chronic pain treatment is for the patient to learn more adaptive coping strategies to deal with the pain experience. For example, if a patient views pain as a punishment, this belief would be addressed, and treatment would focus on challenging the punishment belief and replacing it with a more adaptive view of pain. The patient also needs to learn to accept responsibility for changing his or her behaviors, including lifestyles that may contribute to the pain. This model also focuses on frustrations experienced by the patient.

The Veterans Department of the United States (Murphy et al., 2020) created a cognitive behavioral manual to treat chronic pain, and the authors list the key components of CBT chronic pain program:
   a. Behavioral Activation—increase participation/engagement in rewarding and meaningful activities
   b. Cognitive Restructuring—identify unhelpful/maladaptive thoughts and increase balanced thinking
   c. Relaxation Training—techniques to decrease stress and muscle tension
   d. Pacing—the practice of engaging in an appropriate level of physical activity without significantly increasing pain. By using calculated increases in activity, pacing can lead to greater endurance and a reduced frequency of intensely painful episodes.
   e. Walking—walking program to initiate gradual exposure to movement.
2. Medication Management. Clinicians and physicians must also address the biological component of pain. Pain can be attributed to external trauma and/or from inside the body, such as from the inflammation of joints from osteoarthritis or rheumatoid arthritis. Medication management of pain can reduce or eliminate the signals from the nervous system to the pain centers of the brain. The main treatments for biological pain are over-the-counter medications

(acetaminophen or nonsteroidal anti-inflammatory drugs [NSAIDs] such as ibuprofen and topical sprays) or prescription medications such as nonopioids (e.g., muscle relaxations, anti-anxiety drugs, antidepressants for musculoskeletal pain), stronger pain medications (e.g., codeine), steroid injections, or opioid medication. If opioid medication is prescribed for long-term chronic pain, it is advised that the opioid selection, dosage, duration, follow-up, and discontinuation be closely monitored by the prescribing physician (Murphy et al., 2020). The attending physician must be always assessing risk and abuse of opioid medications. A general rule of thumb is that opioids should *not* be considered first line of therapy for chronic pain for general pain conditions that are not associated with active cancer or palliative or end-of-life care. Physicians should evaluate each patient (age, functional status of patient, etc.) to determine if opioid medication is appropriate and will be of benefit.

3. Stressors. Clinicians and physicians specializing in pain management must address how stress impacts emotional, psychological, physical, and functional factors. There is a relationship between chronic pain and stress. Stress can be broadly defined as a reaction to a challenging emotional or physiological event or series of events resulting in adaptive or maladaptive changes required to regain homeostasis or stability (Sinha & Jastreboff, 2013). Chronic pain may add stress because of reduced income, family tensions, conflicts with employers, and the fear of permanent pain (ACBT, 2020). If there is an increase in emotional/psychological distress with physical arousal, this dynamic can create pain, leading to a cycle of stress-pain-stress, which perpetuates chronic pain and disability (ACBT, 2020).

4. Emotional. Mood is generally impacted when there is limitation placed on well-being. Patients in chronic pain may experience life disruption including, but not limited to, financial distress, loss of friends and social impairment, work limitations or loss of work, functional limitations, and inability to complete activities of daily leading, all of which can negatively impact mood. Chronic pain can lead to depression and loss of motivation, both of which can lead to inadequate effort to recover. If depressed, patients may not feel motivated to seek rehabilitation therapy, go to pain specialists, attend social events, and so on. They may want to stay home and engage in sedentary activity, which can increase pain. Patients can also learn to react adaptively to unpredictable stress that can induced pain (e.g., migraine, headache).

5. Anxiety. There is also accompanying anxiety due to fears of reinjury when pain sufferers attempt to increase activity (ACBT, 2020). The emotional distress can likely cause patients to engage in maladaptive coping (e.g., if I do not move, I will not experience pain).
6. Surgery. Surgical intervention may be warranted to relieve chronic pain, depending on the cause of pain. Patient education about the surgery and recovery period is a necessary part of the treatment plan, and if there will be physical limitations from the surgery, this should also be addressed.

A major decision in treatment planning is addressing the appropriate level of care. The clinician/physicians must choose whether an inpatient or outpatient treatment program would be beneficial for a patient. For patients who are in chronic pain and have additional comorbidities, an inpatient program may be ideal because a multidisciplinary approach to pain may be achieved all in one location. Some individuals may elect to attend outpatient pain treatment programs that may also address a multidisciplinary approach. Clinicians/physicians are encouraged to work with pain specialists who can offer broader treatment plans.

Pain and Sleep

Getting a good night's rest while experiencing pain may not be an easy task. Pain may delay sleep onset and cause sleep disturbance and awakenings, with the result of a decrease in both quality and quantity of sleep. For patients who are sedentary, blood flow to the body is reduced, and when movement occurs, pain and discomfort can also occur. For example, patients with arthritis will experience pain when getting out of bed and walking after waking in the morning.

Pain may alter the position in which patients sleep. Position restriction may occur due to pain; however, movement may occur during the sleep period, causing the patient to experience pain. For instance, if someone breaks an arm and has a cast on it, it may require sleeping in the supine (back) position, and during the night, the person might turn to the side the cast is on, causing pain and awakening.

Chronic Pain and Napping

Napping can occur because the patient was awake most of the night due to pain. resulting in deficient quality and quantity of sleep. If daytime sleepiness occurs, the patient may engage in napping. Depending on the length and timing of the nap, it can interrupt sleep onset and sleep maintenance. Pain medications may also be sedating, which can render chronic pain patients to nap during the day. The full extent that napping has on sleep architecture can be illustrated by thinking of our bodies as a battery. Assume that when we wake up in the morning, our "batteries" are at 100% full, and as the day goes on, the battery is draining. If we nap during the day, our battery is recharged so that we are less likely to fall asleep at our regular bedtime. The result will be delayed sleep and potentially sleep-maintenance interruption.

A 15-minute nap will have less effect on timing of sleep than a two-hour nap. It is also important to look at the time of day or evening that the nap occurs. The closer the nap is to bedtime, the more likely sleep onset will be delayed.

Schaefer et al. (2016) identified a substantial emotional and functional burden on patients. Insomnia and pain are commonly presented in primary care settings (Seng et al., 2016). In Veterans Administration Health facilities, changes in sleep complaints co-occurred with changes in pain complaints. In subsamples of veteran participants where depression screenings verified no depression, the amount of pain was predicted by the quality of sleep (Koffel et al., 2016). In general, pain and insomnia represent common causes for seeking medical care treatment (Karaman et al., 2014).

Development and Causes

The amount of arousal at presleep, including pain discomfort, is a predictor of poor sleep and the development of insomnia (Byers, Lichstein, & Thorn, 2016). The intensity of the pain impacts the patients; views and experiences of their sleep (Gerhart et al., 2017). Covarrubias-Gomez and Mendoza-Reyes (2014) reported that 40% of their sample experienced pain to levels where it impacted their sleep. Depression is a symptom common to posttraumatic stress disorder (PTSD). PTSD and sleep disturbance are significantly associated with pain (Powell et al., 2015). Patients with PTSD indicated higher levels of pain and sleep disturbance than those without PTSD (Powell et al., 2015).

Cognitive perceptions can be influenced by negative mood (Gerhart et al., 2017). Harrison, Wilson, Heron, Stannard and Manafo (2016) identified depressive mood and attention to symptoms as related to heightened ratings of pain and poor sleep. The relationship between pain and sleep is bidirectional, with pain disrupting sleep, and poor sleep accentuating the perception of pain (Harrison et al., 2016).

As stated in chapter 3, the interruption to sleep with leg cramps and leg movements at presleep is problematic. Hoogwout et al. (2015) identified the association between restless leg syndrome and multiple pain problems. The alteration in iron ferritin levels in patients with restless legs syndrome has been suggested as a chemical step in the alteration of dopaminergic metabolism pathways. This pathway is considered to be common to restless legs syndrome, multisite pain, and pain severity (Frange et al., 2014; Hoogwout et al., 2015; Kocabicak et al., 2014).

Yang and Wang (2017) described the chronic pain condition of a migraine as including comorbid conditions that aggravate the pain and contribute to the transition from acute to chronic pain. Sleep disturbance as a comorbid condition to a migraine is experienced in terms of inadequate sleep (Yang & Wang, 2017). Sezgin et al. (2015) described the chronic pain condition of low back pain. Low back pain has been described as commonly located in the lumbar region of the back, bilaterally, with extension of the pain down the legs. The importance of the sleep position (primarily supine position) or extensive time lying and sitting as an attempt to minimize low back pain may actually disturb sleep—both quality and quantity of sleep. While 60–70% of low back pain patients are expected to recover within six weeks, some 10% go on to extensive pain histories lasting for years (Sezgin et al., 2015; Wong, Karppinen, & Samartzis, 2017). Chronic low back pain is considered one of the most common chronic pain conditions that disturbs sleep (Law, Dafton, & Palermo, 2012). Assessment scales such as the McGill Pain Scale are used to gather information about the pain experience from the patient in terms of location, severity, intensity, and type of pain. Mystakidou et al. (2008) identified poor sleep quality in patients with the chronic pain of cancer. The extent of sleep difficulties has been shown to vary with different cancer types (Graci, 2005). For example, one study measuring sleep problems in lung cancer patients, breast cancer patients, insomniacs, and healthy controls found that lung cancer patients had greater decreased sleep efficiency (ratio of time spent sleeping to time spent in bed) compared with breast cancer patients or controls. Lung cancer patients also had longer sleep onset latencies, more fragmented sleep, and more stage 1 sleep (light sleep) than breast cancer patients or controls.

Sexton-Radek, Chami, and Rubinfeld (2017) described the use of antidepressant medications for pain treatment. Use of antidepressant medications is second to pain medication use and contributes to a sedation in dosing schedule that includes presleep to address sleep disturbances in pain patients (Sexton-Radek, Chami, & Rubinfeld, 2017). Specific assessment to determine the patient's perception of his or her pain is essential in pain treatment (Sexton-Radek, 2017; Sexton-Radek & Chami, 2013). However, dosages of pain medication must be carefully monitored given the serious side effects (i.e., respiratory suppression, addiction) (Hassamal, Miotto, Wang, & Saxon, 2016; Morasco, O'Hearn, Turk, & Bobscha, 2014; Yarlas et al., 2015). Alternatives to medication treatment for patients with pain and sleep include cognitive behavior therapy, acupressure, and biofeedback (Gerhart et al., 2017, Graci, 2005; Murphy et al., 2020). Individualized approaches are optimal for those with sleep disturbance and pain (Davin, Wilt, Covington, & Scheman, 2014; Fales, Palermo, Law, & Wilson, 2015; Khusid & Vythilingam, 2016; Yeh et al., 2016).

Effects and Costs

In Society—At Work

The RAND Europe report titled "Why Sleep Matters—the Economic Costs of Insufficient Sleep: A Cross-Country Comparison" identified the United States, compared to the United Kingdom, Japan, Germany, and Canada, as having the highest annual cost of insufficient sleep in gross national product (Hafner, Stepanek, Taylor, Troxel, & Van Stak, 2016). Our country is overspending in medical costs and loss in productivity. When one is experiencing disturbing pain, the pain will interfere with not only quality but also quantity of work performed.

In Society—Up Close

When individuals are sleep deprived from not sleeping well during the night, all aspects of living are affected. Relationships are more likely to be impaired; work performance declines; pain can increase; and individuals are more likely to take time off work/school and cancel social, work, and physical engagements (including doctor appointments).

Case Study: Chronic Low Back Pain and Sleep (Adapted from Graci & Sexton-Radek, 2005)

Ms. Jared was a 54-year-old female presenting with difficulty initiating sleep for at least three of night nights per week over the past month and a lifelong pattern of one night per week. Ms. Jared had been divorced for 17 years, with one disabled adult child in her home and another living independently nearby. She reported a history of thyroid problems, low mood, tinnitus, low back pain, migraines, flu episodes three times a year, and repeated dental procedures (i.e., root canal, crown) the past year. She worked as a high school language teacher. She denied falling asleep while at work, driving, or conversing. She indicated excessive sleepiness in the midafternoon and falling asleep while grading papers in the evening.

A standard sleep interview ruled out sleep disorder. However, she appeared to minimize the level of pain associated with her low back pain during the clinical interview, and in the pain assessment questionnaire, she rated the pain as seven and debilitating. The interview focused on this discrepancy, and Ms. Jared stated that the pain was significant and limited her in most areas of her life.

She was referred to a pain specialist, who recommended physical rehabilitation and NSAID medication. Within two weeks, she reported significant improvement in her low back pain, but when she had to lift her disabled child, the pain returned. By the end of six weeks of physical rehabilitation, she stated that her back felt much stronger, and the pain had significantly diminished. She was also taught how to properly lift a child to avoid low back pain. She also talked to her child's physician about a lifting device as a preventative measure to back pain.

Ms. Jared was also referred for eight sessions of a CBT-focused pain group. Her initial sleep efficiency was 81%, and her final was 86%. Ms. Jared reported relief at the four-week mark, when her sleep restriction plan seemed less intrusive and disruptive, but she would not change her sleep hygiene behaviors (e.g., watching television and reading books before bedtime. For someone who enjoys these activities, they can be mentally stimulating events and can delay sleep onset).

Case Study: Osteoarthritis Pain Management and Sleep
Ms. Gambino is an 86-year-old widowed, retired female who presented with complaints of chronic pain related to osteoarthritis and sleep difficulties related to the pain. She stated that she was diagnosed with osteoarthritis approximately 20 years earlier and that within the last 2 years, her hands, feet, knees, hips, neck, and spine showed signs of significant degenerative joint disease with disfigurement. She could not open her fingers well and could not hold a pen comfortably. She had hypertension as her only medical complaint and was being treated with lisinopril. Other than her osteoarthritis, she was in good health with good reflexes and engaged in most activities unless her pain limited her from going outside her home. She was able to pace her daily activities and enjoyed housecleaning, walking, reading, and watching television. She stated that movement in the morning was unbearable and getting in and out of bed was exceedingly painful. Due to her restriction in

movement and the continual increase in pain, Ms. Gambino stated that she felt like she was getting depressed because "the golden years are not golden at all; pain affects all that I do."

A standard sleep interview ruled out sleep disorder. However, review of her pain assessment revealed that her pain was a 9 out of 10 with the most significant pain occurring in the morning and evening. She stated that her physician had prescribed NSAIDS, but they upset her stomach, and hydrocodone was very sedating. She fell once during the night and would only take it if she were in extreme pain and would then ask that one of her children spend the night with her. Review of her sleep questionnaire revealed that her sleep efficiency was 78% and that she often slept until late morning. She often watched television until between 11:00 p.m. and midnight. She was educated about appropriate sleep hygiene behaviors and was asked to complete a sleep diary/log.

Ms. Gambino was referred to a pain specialist to treat the chronic pain associated with osteoarthritis. Her pain specialist prescribed physical rehabilitation and discussed using cannabidiol (CBD) supplements without tetrahydrocannabinol (THC). She was educated on how CBD works and how it might be beneficial to treat her pain. She stated that she wanted to talk with her children about it but was willing to try the CBD-Biofreeze roll-on medication to treat the pain in her fingers, knees, hips and back. She was asked to return in two weeks.

Review of her sleep diary indicated that she drank one cup of caffeine in the morning, did not eat heavy meals, and did not exercise late in the evening but kept busy throughout the day inside her home unless she was in extreme pain. She tried to "work through" the pain but sometimes it was unbearable. She was instructed to maintain consistent bedtime and wake times, which, at first, she was reluctant to do since she was afraid that if she did not sleep in late during the day that she would get "sick" due to lack of sleep. She was further educated on the principles of sleep and proper sleep hygiene.

Ms. Gambino returned to her pain specialist, and she stated that rehabilitation helped, and the CBD roll-on had been "a life changer" because it "quickly takes away the pain—not all the pain, but it helps." She decided to try the CBD liquid capsules to address a more systemic approach for treatment of her osteoarthritis pain.

She returned two weeks later, and her sleep efficiency score improved to 86%. She stated that it had been very difficult trying to wake up while she still felt sleepy in the morning. She noticed that she was alert more during the day and was in less pain. She saw her pain specialist, and she reported that she had more mobility and that the CBD oil was better than any prescription medication she had tried to date. She did report feeling sleepy during the day, so her CBD dosage was reduced.

Follow-up revealed that her sleep efficiency improved to 91% and that she rated her pain a 4 out of 10 on most days. When she felt her pain was increasing, she started to limit her activity, and this helped. She was consistently going to bed and waking up at the same time and felt like she was a different person. The pain had not gone away, but it was much more manageable. "You learn to live with osteoarthritis, and I have learned how to treat it so that I can live out my golden years."

Case Study

Mr. Anderson was a 33-year-old African American male referred for behavioral counseling. His presenting problem was inability to fall asleep at night due to chronic knee pain. This problem had reportedly occurred since high school (i.e., approximately 18 years ago) when he injured his knee playing football. He stated that his sleep onset was delayed by approximately 30–90 minutes, depending on his pain level. This issue occurred four or five nights per week. The sleep onset difficulty had worsened in the last eight months, with three or more nights per week experiencing a sleep onset delay of two to three hours.

Mr. Anderson worked for Amazon for the last two years. He generally worked the 2–12 shift. His medical history was unremarkable. He described his current sleep onset difficulty as a major stressor and a frustration in his life. He denied depression or anxiety symptoms or the use of prescription or recreational drugs. He denied smoking or drinking. He was of average build and normal weight. He denied napping. He stated that he saw his general practitioner to address the knee pain and she prescribed Motrin for the daily knee pain and Tylenol with codeine for more significant pain. He was currently contemplating knee surgery because he often experienced breakthrough pain with the Motrin, and since he drove a truck for his work, he did not want to take the Tylenol with codeine when he was working.

Mr. Anderson recently bought a condominium and described the home as quiet; he enjoyed watching football, basketball, hockey, golf, and tennis; hiking; and flying his drone. He stated that he had one sister with whom he was close, and they saw each other every Sunday for brunch. He was actively dating and spent weekends with friends.

Mr. Anderson was educated on sleep hygiene, and he agreed to maintain a sleep log. He was also agreeable to attending CBT for chronic pain.

Treatment Summary

Mr. Anderson actively participated in his eight-week CBT program. He stated that throughout the sessions, he was eager to learn ways to cope better with his pain, especially when he couldn't function at 100% while at work. He complied his daily sleep log recordings and all questionnaires for the program. During each session, there was a rotation to each class member reporting how sleep was that past week, and any outstanding experiences related to his or her sleep are queried. He was eager to interact with sleep specialist and the group. Throughout the course, his sleep ratings improved, and his sleep behaviors changed. He repeatedly stated that he experienced frustration when he could not play sports with his friends due to the pain in his knee.

Mr. Anderson complied with all aspects of sleep hygiene and sleep diary completion. He carried his sleep diary/journal with him at all times and recorded pain intensity, type of activity, and mood ratings. His sleep diaries by weeks four and five indicated that he was falling asleep within 30–60 minutes. He was happy with the improvement but wanted to do better. His main challenge was not watching sport recaps before going to bed. He stated that he would get excited or upset, depending how the play went. Class sessions introduced relaxation and guided imagery to help induce relaxation, and he was excited to try this new technique. He was given a DVD to listen to before going to bed.

Mr. Anderson participated in an eight-week CBT sleep class using relaxation techniques. He reported satisfaction at the midpoint and upon completing the class. His final sleep efficiency rating was 94%. Mr. Anderson attributed his success in feeling rested and sleeping well to stopping watching sports before bedtime and engaging in calming presleep activities. Last, he stated that he found a surgeon to repair his knee so that he wouldn't be in chronic pain, but the CBT treatment was beneficial in teaching him how to relax before bedtime and avoid maladaptive sleep hygiene behaviors.

References

ACBT (2020). *Chronic pain*. 54th Annual Convention, November 19–22, Philadelphia, PA, Abstact. http://www.abct.org/Information/?m=mInformation&fa=fs_CHRONIC_PAIN

N. E. Andrews, J. Strong, P. J. Meredith, & R. E. D'Arrigo (2014). Association between physical activity and sleep in adults with chronic pain: A momentary within-person perspective. *Physical Therapy*, 94(4), 499–510.

B. B. Annagur, F. Ugus, S. Apillogullan, T. Kara, & S. Gunduz (2014). Psychiatric disorders and association with quality of sleep and quality of life in patients with chronic pain: A SCID-based study. *Pain Medicine, 15*, 772–781.

J. W. Burns, W. R. Nielson, M. P. Jensen, A. Heapy, R. Czlapinski, R. D. & Kerns (2015). Specific and general therapeutic mechanisms in cognitive-behavioral treatment for chronic pain. *Journal of Consulting and Clinical Psychology, 83*(1), 1–11.

H. D. Byers, K. Lichstein, & B. E. Thorn (2016). Cognitive processes in comorbid poor sleep and chronic pain. *Journal of Behavioral Medicine, 39*, 233–240.

Center for Disease Control (2018). Prevalence of chronic pain and high-impact chronic pain among adults—United States, 2016. *MMWR Morbidity and Mortality Weekly Report, 67*, 1001–1006.

A. Covarrubias-Gomez, & J. J. Mendoza-Reyes (2014). Evaluation of sleep quality in subjects with chronic non-oncological pain. *Journal of Pain & Palliative Care Pharmacotherapy, 27*, 220–274.

S. Davin, J. Wilt, E. Covington, & J. Scheman (2014). Variability in the relationship between sleep and pain in patients undergoing interdisciplinary rehabilitation for chronic pain. *Pain Medicine, 15*, 1043–1051.

J. Fales, T. M. Palermo, E. F. Law, & A. C. Wilson (2015). Sleep outcomes in youth with chronic pain participating in a randomized controlled trial of online cognitive-behavioral therapy for pain management. *Behavioral Sleep Medicine, 13*, 10–123. https://doi.org/10.1080/15402002.2013.8457779

C. Frange, C. Hirotsu, H. Hachul, P. Aranjo, S. Tulik, & M. L. Anderson (2014). Fibromyalgia and sleep in animal models: A current overview and future directions. *Current Pain Headache Reports, 18*, 434. https://doi.org/10.1007/s1916-014-3

J. I. Gerhart, J. W. Burns, K. M. Post, D. A. Smith, L. S. Porter, H. J. Burgess, et al. (2017). Relationships between sleep quality and pain-related factors for people with chronic low back pain: Tests of reciprocal and time of day effects. *Annals of Behavioral Medicine, 51*(3), 365–375.

G. M. Graci (2005). Pathogenesis and management of cancer-related insomnia. *Journal of Supportive Oncology, 3*(5), 349–359.

G. M. Graci, & K. Sexton-Radek (2005). Treatment of sleep disorders using hypnosis and cognitive-behavioral therapies. In R. Chapman (Ed.), *A practitioners case book on CBT and hypnosis* (pp. 349–359). New York: Springer Publications Company.

M. Hafner, M. Stepanek, J. Taylor, W. M. Troxel, & C. Van Stak (2016). *Why sleep matters—The economic cost of insufficient sleep: A cross-country comparative analysis.* New York: Rand Corporation.

L. Harrison, S. Wilson, J. Heron, C. Stannard, & M. R. Manafo (2016) Exploring the association shared by mood, pain-related attention and pain outcomes related to sleep disturbance in a chronic pain sample. *Psychology & Health, 31*(5), 565–577.

S. Hassamal, K. Miotto, T. Wang, & A. J. Saxon (2016). A narrative review: The effects of opioids on sleep disordered breathing in chronic pain patients and methadone maintained patients. *The American Journal on Addictions, 25*, 452–465.

C. S. Hill (2017). Fault lines in familiar concepts of pain. In J. Corns (Ed.), *The Routledge handbook of philosophy of pain* (pp. 1–86). Abingdon: Routledge.

B. M. Hoffman, R. K. Papas, D. K. Chatkoff, & R. D. Kerns (2007). Meta-analysis of psychological interventions for chronic low-back pain. *Health Psychology, 26*(1), 1–9. https://doi.org/10.1037/0278-6133.26.1.1

S. J. Hoogwout, M. V. Paananen, A. J. Smith, D. J. Beales, P. B. O'Sullivan, L. M. Straker, et al. (2015). Mulculoskeletal pain is associated with restless legs syndrome in young adults. *BioMed Central Musculoskeletal Disorders, 16*, 294. https://doi.org/10.1186/s12891-015-0765-1

Institute of Medicine (2006). *Sleep disorders and sleep deprivation: An unmet public health problem*. Washington, DC: The National Academies Press. https://doi.org/10.17226/11617

S. L. James, D. Abate, K. H. Abate, et al. (2018) Global, regional, and national incidence, prevalence, and years lived with disability for 354 diseases and injuries for 195 countries and territories, 1990–2017: A systematic analysis for the Global Burden of Disease Study 2017. *Lancet, 392*: 1789–1858.

S. Karaman, T. Karaman, S. Dogru, Y. Onder, R. Citil, Y. E. Bulut, et al. (2014). Prevalence of sleep disturbance in chronic pain. *European Review for Medical and Pharmacological Science, 18*, 2475–2481.

M. A. Khusid, & M. Vythillingam (2016). The emerging role of mindfulness meditation as effective self-management strategy, Part 2: Clinical implications for chronic pain, substance misuse, and insomnia. *Military Medicine, 181*, 969. https://doi.org/10.725/MLT.MED-D-14-00678

E. Kocabicak, M. Terz, K. Adpinar, K. Paksoy, I. Cebec, & O. Iyigun (2014). Restless legs syndrome and sleep quality in lumbar, radicalapath patients. *Behavioral Neurology, 30*, 245–358.

E. Koffel, K. Kroenke, M. S. Bair, D. Leverty, M. A. Polusny, & E. E. Krebs (2016). The bidirectional relationship between sleep complaints and pain: Analysis of data from a randomized trial. *Health Psychology, 35*(1), 41–49.

E. F. Law, L. Dufton, & T. M. Palermo (2012). Daytime and nighttime sleep patterns in adolescents with and without chronic pain. *Health Psychology, 31*(6), 830–833.

M. A. Lumley, J. L. Cohen, G. S. Borszcz, A. Cano, A. M. Radcliffe, L. S. Porter, et al. (2011). Pain and emotion: A biopsychosocial review of recent research. *Journal of Clinical Psychology, 67*(9), 942–968.

B. J. Morasco, D. O'Hearn, D. Turk, & S. K. Dobscha (2014). Association between prescription opioid use and sleep impairment among veterans with chronic pain. *Pain Medicines, 15*, 1902–1910.

Multiple Chronic Conditions Resource Center (2020). *Chronic pain guidelines*. Retrieved March 18, 2020, from, https://www.multiplechronic conditions.org/chronic-pain-guidelines

J. L. Murphy, J. D. McKellar, S. D. Raffa, M. E. Clark, R. D. Kerns, & B. E. Karlin (2020). *Cognitive behavioral therapy for chronic pain among veterans: Therapist manual*. Washington, DC: U.S. Department of Veterans Affairs, 1–124.

K. Mystakidou, E. Parpa, E. Tsilika, M. Pathiaki, K. Gennatas, V. Smyrniotis, & I. Vassiliou (2007). The relationship of subjective sleep quality, pain and quality of life in advanced cancer patients. *Sleep, 30*(6), 737–742.

National Sleep Foundation (2013). *International bedroom poll summary of findings*. Arlington, VA: National Sleep Foundation.

R. M. Nesse, & P. C. Ellsworth (2009). *Evolution, emotions, and emotional disorders. American Psychologist, 64*, 129–139.

M. A. Powell, V. Corbo, J. R Fonda, J. D. Otis, W. P. Millberg, & R. E. McGlinchey (2015). Sleep quality and reexperiencing symptoms of PTSD are associated with current pain in U.S. OEF/OIF/OND veterans with and without mTBIs. *Journal of Traumatic Stress, 28*, 322–329.

A. Salazaar, M. Duenas, J. A. Mico, B. Ojeda, L. Aguera-Ortiz, J. A. Cervilla, & I. Fallide (2013). Undiagnosed mood disorders and sleep disturbance in primary care patients with chronic musculoskeletal pain. *Pain Medicine, 14*, 1416–1425.

C. Schaefer, R. Mann, E. T. Masters, J. C. Cappelleri, S. R. Daniel, G. Zlateva, et al. (2016). The comparative burden of chronic widespread pain and fibromyalgia in the United States. *Pain Practice, 16*(8), 565–579.

E. K. Seng, C. Cerboni, J. L. Lawson, T. Oken, S. Sheldo, M. D. McKee, & K. A. Bonuck (2016). The burden of sleep problems: A pilot observational study in an ethnically diverse urban primary care setting. *Journal of Primary Care and Community Health, 7*(4), 276–280.

K. Sexton-Radek (2017). Chronic pain pre-surgical assessment and follow-up case study. *Journal of Addiction Research & Therapy, 8*, 5. https://doi.org/10.4172/2155-6105-1000241

K. Sexton-Radek, & A. T. Chami (2013). Pain clinic referral to psychological services best addressed with collaboration. *Health Psychology Research, 1*(3), 173–175.

K. Sexton-Radek, A. Chami & A. Rubinfeld (2017). Pain management strategies: Some uses of antidepressants. *Medications and Nonpharmacological Approaches, 5*, 215–227.

M. Sezgin, E. Z. Hasanefendioglu, M. A. Sungur, N. A. Incel, O. B. Cimon, A. Kanik, & G. Sahin (2015). Sleep quality in patients with chronic low back pain: A cross-sectional study assessing its relation with pain, functional status and quality of life. *Journal of Back and Musculoskeletal Rehabilitation, 28*, 433–441. https://doi.org/10.3233/BMR-140537

R. Sinha, & A. M. Jastreboff (2013). Stress as a common risk factor for obesity and addiction. *Biological Psychiatry, 73*, 827–835.

Y. F. Siu, S. Chan, K. M. Wong, & W. D. Wong (2012). The comorbidity of chronic pain and sleep disturbances in a community adolescent sample: Prevalence and association with sociodemographic and psychological factors. *Pain Medicine, 13*, 1292–1303.

Sleepfoundation.org. (2020) *Pain and sleep*. Retrieved January 2, 2020, from https://www.sleepfoundation.org/articles/pain-and-sleep

S. Sutherland (2017). Rethinking relief. *Scientific American, 3*, 28–35.

J. A. Turner, L. Mancl, & L. A. Aaron (2006). Short- and long-term efficacy of brief cognitive-behavioral therapy for patients with chronic temporomandibular disorder pain: A randomized, controlled trial. *Pain, 121*(3), 181–194.

A. Y. Wong, J. Karppinen, & D. Samartzis (2017). Low back pain in older adults: Risk factors, management options and future directions. *Scoliosis and Spinal Disorders, 12*, 14.

C. P. Yang, & S. J. Wang (2017). Sleep in patients with chronic migraine. *Current Pain Headache Report, 21*, 39. https://doi.org/10.1007/s11916-017-0641-9

A. Yarlas, K. Miller, W. Wen, S. Y. Lynch, S. R. Ripa, J. V. Pergloizzzi, & R. B. Raffa (2015). Buprenorphine transdermal system improves sleep quality and reduces sleep disturbance in patients with moderate-to-severe chronic low back pain: Results from two randomized controlled trials. *Pain Practice, 16*(3), 345–358.

C. H. Yeh, L. K. Suen, J. Shen, L. Chien, Z. Liang, R. M. Glick, et al. (2016). Changes in sleep with auricular point acupressure for chronic low back pain. *Behavioral Sleep Medicine, 14*, 279–294.

CHAPTER 5

Parasomnias

Parasomnias, sleep disorder conditions in which the individual engages in abnormal movement or behaviors that interrupt the sleep cycle, are studied with a routine all-night polysomnogram. For the individual experiencing a parasomnia, it may be frightening, but the parasomnia events are generally benign in nature. Individuals rarely hurt themselves during the parasomnia event. This chapter explores sleep stages as they relate to nonrapid eye movement (NREM) and REM parasomnias, risk factors, and treatment interventions for parasomnias.

In healthy individuals without sleep problems, sleep stages occur in a regular pattern throughout a 24-hour period. Sleep is classified in to two types: dream or REM sleep and NREM sleep. REM sleep occurs every 1.5 hours throughout the sleep interval, which is about 18%–25% of the overall sleep (Graci & Sexton-Radek, 2005). REM periods vary from a few of minutes to an hour plus. REM sleep has a characteristic physiological pattern distinguished by the lateral saccadic rhythm of the eyes, absence of muscle movement, and heightened cardiovascular arousal (Graci & Sexton-Radek, 2005; Sexton-Radek & Graci, 2008). Studies of REM periods by self-report have revealed the changing themes from everyday events to surreal wish fantasies toward the end of the sleep period.

In contrast, NREM sleep occupies a greater portion of the sleep period. NREM is further subdivided into stages 1, 2, 3, and 4, with corresponding physiological activity to each (Graci & Sexton-Radek, 2005). Stage 1 is considered light sleep and is estimated to be some 5% of the sleep period. Stage 2 sleep is about 60% of the sleep intervals and is formally considered "sleep." Stages 3 and 4 are often collapsed together and are classified deep sleep, a physiological event characterized by slow brain wave patterns and increased immune system activity. It is approximately 10–15% of the sleep period.

A night of sleep is characterized as a predicted patterning of sleep onset in 15 minutes, stage 1 sleep onset, and then a progression to stages 2, 3, and 4. On or slightly before 90 minutes after sleep onset, the first REM episode occurs (four to five REM episodes occur per night). Following this, the cycle repeats itself in this progression with four cycles of sleep per night. An excess or deficit in the amount of a type of sleep, a misordering of the timing of sleep, or an intrusion of sleep represents conditions for further study to determine sleep disorder (Graci & Sexton-Radek, 2005).

Parasomnias are divided into three clusters: NREM related, REM related, and other (Sateia, 2014) and may occur at any time during the sleep cycle. Distinguishing between the different types of NREM and REM parasomnias is clinically extremely important because treatment and prognosis may vary (Fleetham & Fleming, 2014). For instance, NREM parasomnias are prevalent in younger individuals and are usually "outgrown" as the person matures into adulthood. REM parasomnias tend to present in late adulthood and are often associated with brain disorders/diseases (American Academy of Sleep Medicine, 2007; American Sleep Disorders Association [ASDA] & American Academy of Sleep Medicine, 2005).

Those sleep events that lead to arousal during REM sleep include REM sleep behavior disorders (RBDs), nightmares, and sleep paralysis (ASDA, 2005; Sateia, 2014; Tinuper, Bisulli, & Provini, 2012). When people enter REM sleep, the body is normally paralyzed to prevent them from acting out their dreams. RBD occurs when people do not remain paralyzed during sleep and may act out their dreams which can cause bodily harm or injury to themselves or their bed partners. Nightmares are often defined as mental experiences that are disturbing in nature and often result in awakenings from sleep (American Academy of Sleep Medicine [AASM], 2007; ASDA & American Academy of Sleep Medicine, 2005). Unfortunately, these mental experiences can evoke feelings of intense fear, terror, or anxiety. Generally, the sleeper can recall the content and details of the nightmare after awakening, and returning to sleep may be difficult. Sleep paralysis can be the frightening experience of waking up or falling asleep when the body is paralyzed for a minute or so, but the mind is awake.

In comparison, those sleep events that lead to partial arousal during NREM sleep include confusional arousals, sleep terrors, and sleepwalking.

Confusional arousals may occur when a person is awakened from stage 3 sleep during the first part of the night (American Academy of Sleep Medicine [AASM], 2013; Graci, 2010; Graci & Sexton-Radek, 2005; Pichardo, 2020). The sleeper has extreme slowness upon awakening and may react slowly to conversations with others or may not understand what someone is trying to communicate. Unlike REM sleep disorders, individuals experiencing confusional arousals may have impaired memory or no recall of the arousal on the following day. Sleep terrors, also referred to as night terrors, occur when a person wakes up with a loud cry or scream and intense feelings of fear (American Academy of Sleep Medicine [AASM], 2007. Often, adults may attempt to escape by jumping from their beds and attempting to leave their bedrooms to go outside. When people are experiencing the intense fear of the sleep terror, they not be responsive to others and can be disoriented and confused, especially if someone tries to awaken them, and they are usually inconsolable. Similar to confusional arousals, people who experience sleep terrors may have no recall of the episode. Last, sleepwalking occurs during NREM sleep (stages 3 and 4), and the person appears to be awake but is asleep and may be moving or appear to be engaged in purposeful behavior. Sleepwalkers do not have memories of the episodes.

There are other parasomnias are not a focus of this chapter. They include sleep-related dissociative disorders, sleep enuresis, sleep-related groaning, exploding head syndrome, sleep-related hallucinations, sleep-related eating disorder, parasomnia unspecified, parasomnia due to drug or substance, and parasomnia due to medical conditions (ASDA & American Academy of Sleep Medicine, 2005; Graci, 2010; Graci & Sexton-Radek, 2005; Sateia, 2014; Tinuper et al., 2012).

Causes

There appears to be a genetic component to parasomnias because parasomnias tend to run in families. Brain disorders may be responsible for some parasomnias—many cases of RBD and RBD are typically seen in males over the age of 50—but they can affect people of all age groups (American Academy of Sleep Medicine, 2007; ASDA & American Academy of Sleep Medicine, 2005; Schenck, 2018). Parasomnias may also be triggered by other sleep disorders, such as obstructive sleep apnea, and by neurologic disorders, such as Parkinson's disease, and by various medications (e.g., antidepressants) or psychiatric diagnoses (e.g., post-traumatic stress disorder [PTSD]) (ASDA & American Academy of Sleep Medicine, 2005; Schenck, 2018). The use of medications with adverse effects related to the central nervous system (e.g., SSRIs, beta blockers, tricyclic antidepressants, and/or sedative hypnotics), nonpharmacological drugs that stimulate the central nervous system (e.g., caffeine, alcohol, nicotine), anxiety, depression, stress, and dementia can also trigger parasomnias (Howell, 2012).

Treatment

Common Parasomnia Treatment Approaches

Treatment for parasomnias involves several components: education, behavioral intervention (e.g., hypnosis, stress management, relaxation/imagery), and, in certain circumstances, medication (Graci & Sexton-Radek, 2005). The first treatment strategy begins with patient education. Patients need to learn how to recognize sleep problems, as well as how they and their provider teams can help them. In the case of parasomnias, the potential for self or bed-partner harm necessitates treatment (Graci, 2010). Education is the key to teaching patients appropriate sleep-hygiene behaviors. Appropriate sleep-hygiene behaviors can include maintaining a regular sleep routine (going to bed and waking up at the same time each day), keeping the home environment safe, and eliminating environmental disturbance (e.g., lights, noises, regulate room temperature, keeping pets out of the bedroom, etc.) (Sexton-Radek & Graci, 2008). Avoiding mentally and physically stimulating activities prior to bedtime (e.g., using social media, surfing the internet) can also significantly impact both sleep quality and quantity. Instead, the sleeper is encouraged to engage in calming, sleep-enhancing behaviors one hour before bedtime and avoiding heavy meals and ingesting of caffeine and alcohol (Graci, 2010).

While including appropriate sleep hygiene into daily and nightly behaviors is important, it is also essential to engage in behaviors that assist in the prevention of parasomnias. For instance, maintaining the same sleep schedule assists in avoiding sleep deprivation, which can trigger some parasomnias. Risk factors for parasomnia include age, genetics, stress, posttraumatic stress disorder, alcohol abuse, drug abuse, medication, and other medical conditions (e.g., REM behavior disorder—acting out dreams while sleeping—is associated with Parkinson's disease) (Schenck, 2018).

Patients are also likely to benefit from the understanding and use of a variety of relaxation techniques (Graci & Sexton-Radek, 2005). These range from relatively simple techniques that require three to five minutes of instruction to much more complex shifts in the patients' view of life, which consume two months or more of teaching. Some of these techniques may include guided imagery, progressive muscle relaxation, and biofeedback.

Cognitive behavioral therapy may be used with efficacious outcomes that primarily focus on alleviating the fear, terror, and anxiety that may be related to the parasomnia. Generally, cognitive behavioral therapy is a long-term strategy and may be used in conjunction with hypnosis, relaxation techniques, and medication management. If the individual does not respond to education and behavioral management approaches, a more thorough pharmacological approach may be warranted, and the patient should consult with a physician. Treatment can be efficacious if the patient begins medication management.

The most common parasomnias that have been amenable to hypnosis/ hypnotherapy include nightmare, sleep terror, sleepwalking, and night eating disorder (Sharma, 2007). Other parasomnias may be treated with hypnosis; however, treatment efficacy is lacking. Those sleep disorders with an organic or medical basis associated with them (e.g., REM sleep behavior disorder) may still be treated with hypnosis for the benefits of relaxation and stress management.

Clinical hypnosis is a safe and effective method of treating certain parasomnias because it allows the clinician to gain access to the underlying problem (Graci, 2010; Modlin, 2002). It may also be considered a tool that can be utilized to amplify the therapeutic effects of therapy (Ng & Lee, 2008). Self-hypnosis is considered a voluntary relaxation technique (Kryger, 2004) that is like meditation in that it can ease the body and mind into preparing for sleep (Hammond, 1990). Hypnosis and self-hypnosis offer rapid methods to managing anxiety and worry often associated with stressors, facilitating deep relaxation and controlling mental overactivity and decreasing physiological arousal (Graci & Sexton-Radek, 2005; Hammond, 1990; Kryger, 2004). Hypnosis has been found to be effective in reducing stress and promoting relaxation, which may or may not cause a reduction in sleep disturbance episodes. If it is determined that the parasomnias have a psychological contributor (e.g., nightmares, sleep walking episodes related to a traumatic injury), they are very amenable to hypnotism.

The key element in treating sleep disorders of this kind is essentially symptom reduction and not cure. It is also important to consider whether the side effects of medications produce parasomnia symptoms, in which case, hypnosis is unlikely to have a therapeutic effect.

From a pharmacological (medication management) perspective, the use of antidepressants or benzodiazepine medications may be used in the treatment of parasomnias. While these medications may reduce parasomnia episodes, they can be used to increase quality and quantity of sleep. Benzodiazepines (e.g., clonazepam) and antidepressants (e.g., amitriptyline) will be taken prior to sleep, and melatonin is taken several hours before bedtime (*Best Practice Journal*, 2012). For those individuals at risk for falls (e.g., the elderly), benzodiazepines may not be safe and should be prescribed with caution. In this case, alternative medication management should be explored.

While most parasomnias may not be harmful (although frightening), keeping the environment safe is exceedingly important. For cases where the individuals are a threat to themselves or other members of a household, medication management will be the first line of treatment.

Behavioral and cognitive behavioral treatment approaches are initially more time-consuming and more expensive than medications. However, over the life span, with total physician visits and prescriptions, it may be more cost-effective for patients to engage in behavioral and cognitive behavioral treatments if the parasomnia disorder is responsive to treatments.

Effects and Costs

In Society

Parasomnias can have a negative effect on people's lives and reduce their quality of life. People may act in bizarre, unusual, or violent behavior, but parasomnias are rarely linked to mental disorders. However, people who suffer from parasomnias may endure ridicule, confusion, or shame about their symptoms (Schenck, 2018). These feelings or experiences may lead to avoidance of social or emotional interactions with others. However, for those who experience parasomnias, improvement in their symptoms can be improved with good sleep habits. Many people who suffer with parasomnias see an improvement in their symptoms simply by improving their sleep habits. Medical intervention may be needed to evaluate and treat parasomnia episodes when there is risk of injury or harm to oneself or another person due to the parasomnia (Fleetham & Fleming, 2014).

When children experience parasomnias, they will most likely stop occurring with age. For parasomnias associated with drugs, alcohol, medications, stress, and so on, the parasomnia events will most likely cease once the stressors or drugs/alcohol/medications are terminated.

In Relationships

Both the person experiencing the parasomnia episodes and the bed partner can have disturbed sleep. The disturbed sleep can strain relationships for a variety of factors. The bed partner may fear sleeping with someone who has parasomnias for fear of getting injured or losing of sleep. In many cases, seeking help from a therapist or support group can help people with parasomnias and the people close to them cope with these issues. Untreated parasomnias can lead to relationship deterioration because witnessing a parasomnia from the bed partner's perspective can be frightening. Loss of sleep can impact not only the relationship but also the work performance of either or both sleepers. The bed partner can become anxious about the potential to lose sleep while contemplating if the partner will experience a parasomnia. When sleep intervention is sought, the outcomes of loss of sleep for either the patient or bed partner will decrease.

At Work

If sleep is disturbed during the night and sleepiness occurs the day, a person is a risk for injury, loss of employment, absenteeism, and low performance ratings. If experiencing disturbed sleep during the night and experiencing daytime sleepiness, caution must be exercised if engaging in work that requires vigilance (e.g., handling heavy machinery, driving a truck) for risk of injury or death. People perform at their best when they feel rested, and if parasomnia episodes/events are impacting sleep quality and quantity, seeking medical care is necessary to explore the sleep disturbance and appropriate treatment options.

Once the patient has been educated and is implementing adaptive sleep-hygiene behaviors, sleep-restriction therapy, stimulus control therapy, or cognitive therapy, induction, deepening, and then hypnotic suggestions may be implemented. The following examples are posthypnotic suggestions to be used for parasomnia treatment (adapted from Graci, 2010).

You will experience feelings of safety and security during sleep and return safely to bed.

Your sleep will be restful sleep, with minimal movement or awakenings.

When your feet touch the floor, you will awaken feeling calm and peaceful and return safely to bed.

When you touch your doorknob or the lock on your door, you will awaken feeling calm and peaceful. You will calmly and safely return to bed.

When you touch your window, you will awaken feeling calm and peaceful and return safely to bed.

When you touch your refrigerator door, you will awaken feeling calm and peaceful and return safely to bed.

The reader is cautioned that not all patients are suggestive, so the impact of hypnosis on sleep change is variable. Hypnosis will promote feelings of relaxation and may be used as a powerful tool for presleep relaxation. The benefits of relaxation are effective on sleep.

Despite the lack of research on the effects of hypnosis on the treatment of parasomnias, there is agreement that hypnosis is a noninvasive, inexpensive, side-effect free, short-term treatment for the treatment of parasomnias (Graci & Sexton-Radek, 2005; Hauri, Silber, & Boeve, 2007; Kennedy, 2002; Ng & Lee, 2008; Quan, 2006). Furthermore, hypnotherapy allows unconscious exploration of underlying functions and conflicts associated with the sleep disturbance (Hammond, 1990).

The following cases represent an amalgamation of cases and groups that have been treated using the concepts, assessments, and treatments for parasomnias (adapted from Graci, 2010). Two case examples are discussed.

Case Study 1

Mrs. Jones is a 26-year-old Caucasian female referred for a sleep consult by her psychologist. Her presenting problem was frequent nocturnal arousals in which she would sit up in bed with her feet resting on the floor and begin to yell, scream, grab her throat, and experience shortness of breath with intense feelings of terror. She reported that when these events occurred, she believed that she was dying, and she could not be consoled by any member of her family. Mrs. Jones denied remembering what caused the sleep arousal or the content of her dream. She brought two videos to the session which captured these "episodes."

Mrs. Jones had been married for eight years and had four children, aged one, three, five, and six. Her sleep arousal problems were reported to occur for the last three years. However, the frequency and intensity of these sleep awakenings increased over time. A thorough sleep evaluation was conducted, and the following information was collected. She reported no difficulty falling asleep; however, during the week, she frequently experienced early morning awakenings with an inability to return to sleep. She had a slender body habitus and her physical exam was negative for a diagnosis of sleep apnea.

Mrs. Jones was a full-time homemaker and home schooled her children. She stated that she loved her husband and children. However, she always wanted to earn her college degree, but with the pregnancy and birth of each child, she stated that she realized this "dream" was never going to come to fruition. She portrayed herself as daydreamer, often daydreaming about what it would be like to attend college, graduate with a psychology degree, and possibly attend graduate school so that she could become a psychologist.

She described her husband as a dedicated husband and father who worked long hours as an engineer. Mrs. Jones repeatedly stated that she shared her "dreams" of attending college with her husband before they were married and during their marriage, but he did not support her them. He told her that being a wife and mother is the most "noble" profession and she should not want anything more. Mr. Jones is the main financial contributor to the family, and he told her that they have everything they could need or want because he "provides for his family." Overall, Mrs. Jones stated that she enjoyed her life but rarely had energy or time for personal or social interests (e.g., private time, going out with friends). She also stated that, at times, she felt as though she were "suffocating" because she had so much work to do during the day and night.

Mrs. Jones's medical history was unremarkable. She was unable to provide an explanation for her arousals from sleep and voiced significant upset and frustration with these events. She stated that she was beginning to fear falling asleep at night because when these events occurred, they were so frightening that she would remain awake for several hours until she calmed down and relaxed. She denied symptoms of depression or the use of drugs but endorsed experiencing anxiety because she had so much to do accomplish daily and often did not get everything done that she needed to for the day. She denied drinking or smoking. She stated that she used to exercise but stopped after the birth of her second child because of time constraints. Mrs. Jones reported nightly bedtimes between 10:30 and 11:00 p.m., and her reported wake-up time was 6:00–6:30 a.m. daily. She endorsed sleepiness during the day but denied napping.

Mrs. Jones lived in a two-story home with her family and mother- and father-in-law. She stated that her in-laws are somewhat demanding, but the relationship is "good." Her hobbies include reading, watching television, and taking walks. She indicated that she often does not have time for hobbies.

Mrs. Jones was unfamiliar with relaxation techniques; she indicated receptivity to learning hypnosis and to the logging of her sleep.

Summary

After a thorough sleep intake and assessment, Mrs. Jones was diagnosed with sleep terror disorder. Treatment included two sessions of hypnosis and continued work with her psychologist.

In the first session, she indicated a willingness to "learn new things" and was attentive during the session. She complied with daily sleep-log recordings. During hypnosis, she was asked how she felt emotionally during the day, and she replied, "I feel like I am being suffocated because I am so busy, and there is no time for me." Mrs. Jones stated that she felt relaxed after the session, but home practice was not as relaxing. Hypnotic suggestions included falling into a deep sleep and maintaining this deep sleep throughout the night (unless she had to use the bathroom); if awakened, she would feel safe and secure, and return to sleep would be easy. Suggestions also included that when she awakened and her feet touched the floor, she would awaken feeling calm and peaceful. Breathing would be slow and unlabored. She would take oxygen in and out of her lungs easily.

It was apparent that Mrs. Jones felt suffocated in her daytime life (performing motherly duties, homeschooling her children, cleaning and cooking, taking care of her in-laws, and having to give up her dreams of attending college) and acted out these feelings in her sleep-terror episodes. After two sessions, her sleep diary indicated that she was sleeping better, and the frequency of these arousal episodes had significantly declined. Mrs. Jones's psychologist continued to assist her in processing her conflicted feelings of being a mother and wanting to accomplish her dreams and goals. Within a year, Mrs. Jones denied having sleep-terror episodes.

Case Study 2

Ms. Tyler was a 38-year-old female presenting with sleepwalking episodes and nocturnal binge-eating episodes. These episodes occurred approximately three times per week, and their initial onset began 6 years ago. Ms. Tyler was single and employed as a secretary. She had been involved in an on-again, off-again intimate relationship with her significant other for the last 4 years. She described herself as an attention-to-detail person and enjoyed her job. She had an active social life, attending social events with friends several times a week. Ms. Tyler was an avid cyclist and biked approximately 60 miles per week. She stated that biking was her primary stress release, and she looked forward to biking daily. Furthermore, Ms. Tyler described herself as a restrictive eater, primarily eating low-fat, low-carbohydrate food. She stated that she enjoyed having dessert occasionally and made sure that "she makes up for indulging" with her next biking session. She denied a significant medical history but endorsed experiencing mild depression for the last 20 years and had been in psychotherapy for 6 years. She stated that she enjoyed the "supportive component" of therapy. Ms. Tyler was a tall, slender woman and denied experiencing symptoms of apnea, periodic leg movement disorder, restless leg syndrome, or sleep paralysis.

A standard sleep interview indicated that during her sleepwalking episodes, she had walked out of her home (she lived in a high-rise condominium), telephoned friends in the middle of the night, and written emails. She repeatedly stated that she was embarrassed by these nightly behaviors, especially the nonsensical emails. Furthermore, she stated that during some of her sleepwalking events, she would go to her refrigerator and eat frozen leftovers. Ms. Tyler had also eaten entire frozen entrées with no recollection the following morning, except the feeling of abdominal "fullness." She would find the empty food containers in the trash with no other visible evidence that she ate during the night. Ms. Tyler denied a childhood history of sleepwalking or sleep talking.

Prior to going to bed, Ms. Tyler engaged in mentally stimulating activities and often had work issues on her mind. Typically, she fell asleep within 30 minutes, but within two to three hours after sleep onset, she engaged in sleepwalking/sleep eating episodes. These episodes occurred two or three times per week.

Ms. Tyler was diagnosed with a sleepwalking disorder. Treatment was formulated from the information gathered during the intake, and hypnotic suggestions were generated from this information.

Ms. Tyler was seen for two sessions. The first session included hypnotic suggestions for when her feet touched the floor, when she touched her laptop cover, when she touched the doorknob to her bedroom door, and when she opened the refrigerator door, she would awaken feeling calm and safe and would return to bed. Suggestions for maintaining a deep and restorative sleep (with minimal movement) throughout the night were also given to Ms. Tyler. This first session also included education on maintaining proper sleep-hygiene behaviors. For instance, she was instructed not to exercise for at least four hours before bedtime, avoid sleep deprivation, avoid mentally stimulating activities at least one hour prior to bedtime, and so on. After the first session, she reported a significant decrease in sleepwalking/eating episodes with continued decline after the second session (she reported experiencing one sleepwalking/sleep eating episode for the month). Ms. Tyler continued to see her therapist and work on issues related to "the need to feel in control" and learn more effective methods for coping with stress(ors). Her therapist began to focus on the conscious and unconscious causes for her sleep disturbance.

References

American Academy of Sleep Medicine (2007). *International classification of sleep disorders: Diagnostic and coding manual* (2nd ed.). Westchester, IL: American Academy of Sleep Medicine.

American Academy of Sleep Medicine (2013). An overview of parasomnias. In *Diagnostic and statistical manual of mental disorders, 5th edition: DSM-5*. Arlington, VA: American Psychiatric Association.

ASDA, & American Academy of Sleep Medicine (2005). *The international classification of sleep disorders: Diagnostic and coding manual* (2nd ed.). Westchester, IL: American Academy of Sleep Medicine.

H. Attarian (2010). Treatment options for parasomnias. *Neurologic Clinics, 28*(4), 1089–1106.

J. Fleetham, & J. Fleming (2014). Parasomnias. *CMAJ, 186*(8), E273–E280.

G. Graci (2010). Hypnotherapy and parasomnias. In M. J. Thorpy & G. Plazzi (Eds.), *The Parasomnias and other sleep-related movement disorders* (pp. 338–344). Cambridge, MA: Cambridge University Press.

G. M. Graci, & K. Sexton-Radek (2005). Treating sleep disorders using cognitive behavioral therapy and hypnosis. In R. A. Chapman (Ed.), *The clinical use of hypnosis in cognitive behavior therapy: A practitioner's casebook* (p. 348). New York: Springer Publishing Company.

D. Hammond (1990). Sleep disorders. In *Handbook of hypnotic suggestions and metaphors* (pp. 220–221). New York: W.W. Norton.

P. Hauri, M. Silber, & B. Boeve (2007). The treatment of parasomnias with hypnosis: A 5-year follow-up study. *Journal of Clinical Sleep Medicine, 15*(3[4]), 369–373.

M. J. Howell (2012). Parasomnias: An updated review. *Neurotherapeutics, 9*, 753–775.

G. A. Kennedy (2002). A review of hypnosis in the treatment of parasomnias: Nightmare, sleepwalking, and sleep terror disorders. *Australian Journal of Clinical and Experimental Hypnosis, 30*(2), 99–155.

M. Kryger (2004). *A woman's guide to sleep disorders* (1st ed.). New York: McGraw-Hill.

T. Modlin (2002). Sleep disorders and hypnosis: To cope or cure? *Sleep & Hypnosis, 4*(1), 39–46.

G. Pichardo (2020). Parasomnias. *WebMD*. Retrieved May 31, 2021, from https://www.webmd.com/sleep-disorders/parasomnias

B.-Y. Ng, & T.-S. Lee (2008). Hypnotherapy for sleep disorders. *Annals of the Academy of Medicine, Singapore, 37*, 683–688.

S. Quan (2006). Podcast of the Journal of Clinical Sleep Medicine. *Journal of Clinical Sleep Medicine, 1*(2), 1–3.

M. J. Sateia (2014). International classification of sleep disorders-third edition: Highlights and modifications. *Chest, 146*(5), 1387–1394 from https://www.sleepfoundation.org/articles/sleep-and-parasomnias

K. Sexton-Radek, & G. Graci (2008). *Combatting Sleep Disorders* (1st ed.). Westport, CT: Praeger Publishers, p. 152.

S. Sharma, S. Hadigal, M. Wagner, S. Ryals, & R. S. Berry (2007). Patient with a new parasomnia. *Journal of Clinical Sleep Medicine, 15*(6), 929–930.

P. Tinuper, F. Bisulli, & F Provini (2012). The parasomnias: Mechanisms and treatment. *Epilepsia, 53*(Suppl. 7), 12–19.

CHAPTER 6

Narcolepsy

Theory and Research

The neurological condition of narcolepsy typically emerges between the ages of 10 and 20. In some groupings of people, a genetic lineage has been identified, but this is not the case for everyone. Other species, including dogs, can suffer from this condition. Narcolepsy affects many aspects of quality of life for patients diagnosed and living with it. However, many narcoleptic patients, when adequately treated, can live normal lives. This chapter will focus on the medical facts regarding narcolepsy as well as its impact on quality of life.

Risk factors for narcolepsy include age and family history. Narcolepsy can occur at any age; however, it is more common to be diagnosed between the ages of 10 and 30. Those with a family history of narcolepsy have about a 20–40 times greater risk of a narcolepsy diagnosis than those without a family history of narcolepsy (Mayo Clinic, 2019). Additionally, people who are diagnosed with narcolepsy tend to be overweight.

The core symptoms of narcolepsy are excessive daytime sleepiness, sleep paralysis, and cataplexy. Cataplexy is characterized as a state of muscle atonia which causes the individual to not be supported and consequently fall. A particularly problematic expression of these symptoms is the frequent sleep attacks. Sleep attacks can last from seconds to minutes and are prompted by neurological triggers related to midbrain functioning, such as emotion, muscle fatigue, or neuron misfiring.

In narcoleptic patients, sleep paralysis occurs at the start and stop of sleep. Sleep paralysis is characterized by feelings of dread and fear (e.g., as if an intruder is in the bedroom). Research in this area has defined the sleep paralysis as related to misfiring or missignaling of neurons involved in rapid eye movement (REM) dream sleep (Olunu et al., 2018). Muscle atrophy, sometimes called "paralysis," co-occurs with sleep paralysis. Patients with narcolepsy report that the paralysis occurring along with the confusing state of REM-like activity together make the fear particularly dreadful and frightening.

While not all patients with narcolepsy experience cataplexy (reports suggest that about 70% do), the symptom is particularly frightening (Schiappa, Scarpelli, D'Atri, Gorgoni, & L. De Gennaro, 2018). Patients with both narcolepsy and cataplexy experience muscle atonia and weakness to the extent that they collapse. Patients are usually amnesic to these cataplexic episodes. The term cataplexy comes from *kata* (Greek) for down and *plexis* meaning a stroke or seizure (De la Herrán Arita, Alberto, Equihua-Benítez, & Drucker-Colin, 2013). The cataplexic attacks are triggered by strong emotions and muscle sensations, such as standing for too long, or a combination of these, such as sitting in the bath— the combination of the immobility of the legs and pleasurable sensation of the warm water. Equally perplexing is the patient's amnesia of the cataplexic attack. Interestingly, even during sleep, narcolepsy-cataplexy patients tend to have different emotional experiences than healthy control subjects, with more vivid, bizarre, and frightening dreams (Olunu et al., 2018).

Emotional functioning and narcolepsy have a dysregulation that occurs such that emotions can trigger cataplexy. Olunu et al. (2018) state that some symptoms of narcolepsy depend on emotional stimuli. For example, emotional inputs, such as laughing, joking, or anger, can trigger cataplectic attacks, as can a pleasant surprise. The authors further state that neurophysiological and neurochemical findings suggest the involvement of emotional brain circuits in the physiopathology of cataplexy, which seems to depend on the dysfunctional interaction between the hypothalamus and the amygdala that is associated with an alteration of hypocretin levels. Unfortunately, the relationship between emotion and narcolepsy has been poorly investigated.

The midbrain structure called the hypothalamus conveys brain stem and cortex signals. In patients with narcolepsy, the reception and conveyance to turn off continued function and turn on sleep function is misgauged. The hypothalamus deregulation also results in a nontypical sleep architecture. The sleep state is different for the narcoleptic patient. The amount of time to enter full sleep, including how the narcolepsy patient enters and exits sleep, is qualitatively different compared to health controls (Scammell & Winrow, 2011). The chemical orexin has been identified as irregular in narcoleptic patients. Furthermore, the role of orexin in the hypothalamic regulation of sleep-wake state. Scientific investigation in this area has identified orexin deficits and erratic, nontypical sleep in narcolepsy.

Normal sleep architecture begins with nonrapid eye movement (NREM) and cycles through different sleep stages, including REM; however, in narcoleptic sleep, the patient may enter REM sleep suddenly, without first experiencing NREM sleep. This sudden entry into REM sleep can occur during the day or night. Some of the characteristics of narcolepsy, including cataplexy, sleep paralysis, and hallucinations, are similar to changes that occur in REM sleep, but they occur during wakefulness or drowsiness (Mayo Clinic, 2019).

Currently, narcolepsy is subdivided into two types according to the *International Classification of Sleep Disorders*, 3rd edition: narcolepsy type 1 (NT1) and narcolepsy type 2 (NT2) (American Academy of Sleep Medicine [AASM], 2014). NT1 has the distinctive features of excessive daytime sleepiness, cataplexy, hypnagogic hallucinations, and sleep paralysis and is caused by a marked reduction in neurons in the hypothalamus that produce orexin (hypocretin), which is a wakefulness-associated neuropeptide (American Academy of Sleep Medicine [AASM], 2014). NT2 has the distinctive features of NT1, except for cataplexy. Patients with narcolepsy and cataplexy (NT1) carry the HLA-DQB1*0602 haplotype, which is a disease-modifying allele (Watson, Ton, Koepsell, Gersuk, & Longstreth, 2010). NT2 is a complex disorder, and its genetic sequencing is poorly understood.

For those patients who experience cataplexy, education is the key to encountering emotional triggers. Situations involving joking, laughing, or even tickling can trigger cataplexy. Family and friends are encouraged to avoid these triggers or situations (Mayo Clinic, 2019). Avoiding strong emotions may seem unpleasant; however, decreasing episodes of cataplexy may outweigh the negativity of avoiding strong emotions. People can learn to "tone down" their emotions so that information is not perceived as "strong," thus lessening the chance of a cataplexic event from occurring.

Most diagnosed narcoleptics (Doghramji, Lieberman, & Gordon, 2007) experience excessive daytime sleepiness (EDS). Patients with narcolepsy fall asleep without warning, at any time and in any place. For instance, narcoleptic patients might be working or talking with friends and suddenly nod off. They can even fall asleep while standing up. One may see how narcoleptic patients can be easily injured and should avoid working with dangerous equipment or machinery, even if there is only a slight chance of nodding off while working. They can sleep for a few minutes or up to 30 minutes, and they feel refreshed upon awakening but may then fall asleep again (Mayo Clinic, 2019).

The prevalence of narcolepsy in the United States is approximately 1 in 2,000 people. Prevalence figures are higher in Japan—some 1 per 600 population (Doghramji et al., 2007). Patients with narcolepsy are at risk of falling asleep in situations that will put them at risk (e.g., while driving or standing in line at the store). Consequently, the narcoleptic patient's lifestyle becomes circumscribed to avoid the detrimental effects that may happen with sleep attacks. When patients experience sleep attacks, they may experience ridicule from friends who do not understand the disorder. These negative perceptions can have detrimental psychological consequences on narcoleptic patients—they may be ostracized from social circles and feel like an outcast. Keeping a job may be difficult because they often feel sleepy, and school or work performance may decline.

Patients taking antidepressants may experience sleepiness because some antidepressants have sedating properties and can increase daytime sleepiness. Additionally, patients with cataplexy have the most compromised lifestyles. Last, narcoleptic patients with cataplexy are at a greater risk of developing REM behavior disorder (Nevisimalova et al., 2013). Some 70,000 hypothalamic neurons responsible for generating orexin are lost in individuals with narcolepsy with cataplexy (Mahoney, Cogswell, Koralnik, & Scammell, 2019).

Gupta, Shulda, Goyal, Srivastava, and Bihari (2012) report that of their narcolepsy clinic patients, 60% had cataplexy, and 15% of these patients experienced accidents, including those that were life-threatening. Peacock and Benca (2010) emphasized the need for distinguishing symptoms and behavior of narcolepsy from major depressive disorder, bipolar disorder, and psychotic disorders. An all-night polysomnogram followed by a multiple sleep latency test (MSLT), physical exam, and psychological assessment is essential to a correct diagnosis of narcolepsy (Dunne, Patel, Maschauer, Morrison, & Riha, 2016; Melamed, Delayahu, & Palgacu, 2009; Mysliwiec & Brock, 2018). Bladin (2000) emphasized the need to address emotional factors related to narcolepsy in patients to assist them with their adjustment to the condition. Kim et al. (2009) reported reduced gray matter volume in the right hypothalamus. Kim et al. (2009) examined variations of narcolepsy by clinical evaluation and reported more similarities between narcolepsy and cataplexy and idiopathic hypersomnia. Idiopathic hypersomnia patients experience varying levels of disrupted sleep and excessive daytime sleepiness. From clinical evaluation, Bahammam (2007) identified that narcoleptic patients with cataplexy have a higher incidence of periodic leg movements (PLM) during their sleep (i.e., rhythmical extensions of the great toe and partial flexion of the ankle, knee, and hip that lasts 0.5–5 seconds). Pizza, Tartarott, Poryazova, Bauman, and Bassetti (2013) conducted both clinical evaluations and polysomnogram (PSG)/MSLT and found a comorbidity of narcolepsy with cataplexy and PLM as well as narcolepsy with cataplexy and sleep apnea.

Treatment

Behavioral strategies and therapy in combination with medication are the ideal treatment plan for narcolepsy. Medications allow the narcoleptic patient to feel and act more alert. Behavioral strategies can also increase alertness. These include daytime napping and staying active to keep alert. Napping may feel refreshing, and the patient may experience improved alertness for one to three hours postnap (Harvard Medical School, 2019). The key element is that patients need to limit naps to 15–20 minutes (power naps) because sleeping longer can interrupt nocturnal sleep. Patients should schedule consistent daytime naps at the time they find it the most difficult to stay awake. Some narcoleptic patients find it difficult to stay awake in the midafternoon (two to three o'clock), and if severe sleepiness occurs, they can schedule an additional nap in the late morning (Harvard Medical School, 2019). Additionally, to ensure alertness, taking a nap before driving may be beneficial. For most other types of sleep disorders and diagnoses (e.g., insomnia) patients should avoid napping because it will interfere with nighttime sleep. In addition, engaging in healthy sleep-hygiene behaviors can positively impact narcoleptic sleep. Caffeine and exercise in the evening will interfere with sleep. Last, sedating medications (e.g., allergy medication) and heavy meals can cause delays in sleep onset. Patients are encouraged to discuss taking sedating medications with their physicians to determine if another type of medication can be substituted or if the timing of the medication can be moved.

The pharmaceuticals primarily prescribed are amphetamines, which treat the symptom of excessive daytime sleepiness. Antidepressant medications are prescribed to suppress REM and to treat the nontypical sleep pattern with REM onset and sleep paralysis.

Effects and Costs

In society. Patients with narcolepsy, if employed, worry about the security of their positions. Also, given the medical costs of the condition (i.e., medication, annual PSG/MSLT) the chronic nature of narcolepsy draws from the economy to some extent.

At work. Given the symptoms of narcolepsy, functioning successfully at a vocation is quite difficult, but patients do not qualify for social security disability income. Some may be able to list cognitive seizures as a type of epilepsy, which sometimes qualifies for disability. Additionally, the excessive daytime sleepiness results in four to five hours of drowsiness during the day, preventing the individual from working. There is no documentation of the socioeconomic impact, in general, of narcolepsy. However, there are vocational restrictions for narcoleptics, such as working with heavy machinery, driving, or doing any task that requires vigilance. If a child wants to become a pilot and is then diagnosed with narcolepsy, this diagnosis can be seen as a shattering of dreams.

In relationships. Patients with narcolepsy typically experience impactful changes in their relationships. If employed, patients are worried about loss of their job due to EDS. Adolescent and young adult patients feel embarrassed and ashamed about their pervasive disorder. In adults, marital difficulties are common. Often, narcoleptic patients are not allowed to drive due to potential injury to themselves or others if they were to fall asleep while behind the wheel. Narcoleptic patients may also feel stigmatized, as maintaining relationships may be difficult due to the changes in lifestyle that are required to manage the narcolepsy.

Case Study: Sleep-Related Hallucinations, Confusional Arousals, and REM Behavior Disorder in Narcolepsy

John is a 19-year-old college student who was diagnosed with narcolepsy at 18 years old. He stated that when he was 16 years old, he often fell asleep during class and experienced excessive daytime sleepiness. As he matured, the symptoms became worse, and he would "fall asleep while standing, eating talking with someone." One day, he was driving to school one morning, fell asleep at the wheel, and sideswiped his car with another car. He was brought to the emergency room and, with additional testing and an overnight sleep study, a diagnosis of narcolepsy was given to John. He is not allowed to drive and has difficulty getting restful sleep at night. Prior to treatment for narcolepsy, he reported experiencing sleep hallucinations that were frightening and he acted out his dreams a couple of times. On one occasion, he fell out of bed and injured his arm. He has returned to school and presented for clinical intervention to learn strategies for dealing with the stress associated with a diagnosis of narcolepsy. He stated that since he cannot drive, he must either rely on friends for transportation or take the city bus. He has difficulty keeping a job because he still experiences daytime sleepiness. He wants to "feel normal" in a world that does not understand narcolepsy, and at his age, it impacts his quality of life.

He needs to maintain a strict sleep-and-wake schedule, and as a college student, he often has to turn down events. On the occasions when he stays out late with friends, he is sleep deprived, and this aggravates the narcolepsy. People often make fun of him if he has a sleep attack because they do not understand the features and clinical signs of narcolepsy. He stated that he is tired of being the butt of people's jokes. He also stated that he feels like "a ninety-year-old man trapped in a young man's body."

While John engages in healthy sleep-hygiene behaviors and has a strict sleep-and-wake routine, he wants to learn additional techniques to assist him in coping more adaptively with narcolepsy. Therapy focused on not only supportive therapy but also cognitive behavioral therapy to address his beliefs that narcolepsy is ruining his life. Part of his therapy assignments was to explore the things in life that narcolepsy does not limit him to.

He was initially only able to focus on the limitations of narcolepsy. After four sessions, he developed some insight that he is still able to enjoy going to the movies; playing video games; and spending time with family, friends, and girlfriends. He likes the taste of coffee, so he has learned to drink decaffeinated coffee. If he needs to go somewhere and a friend cannot drive him, he can take a taxi or ridesharing service (even though there is a higher cost associated with this type of transportation than with the city bus).

He was asked to keep a sleep log and food diary for two weeks. When reviewed, his sleep schedule was more variable than what he stated. For instance, he stated that his bedtime was between 10:30 and 11:00 p.m. and that his wake times between 8:00 and 8:30 a.m., but he recorded sleep bedtimes between 10:30 p.m. and 1:00 a.m., with wake times between 10:00 and 11:00 a.m. When queried about his sleep schedule, he stated that he plays video games, and when he is enjoying the game, he sometimes stays up later than expected.

Therapy focused on maintaining sleep and wake times. He agreed to stop playing video games by 9:00 p.m. and participate in relaxing and nonstimulating activities. He stated that reading makes him sleepy and listening to jazz music relaxes him, so he was encouraged to engage in both activities. He was instructed not to text, use the internet, or watch movies or television because these activities are mentally stimulating. He agreed and completed another two weeks of sleep logs.

Review of his sleep logs revealed that he was adhering to the treatment plan, and he reported feeling less sleepy during the day and slightly more energetic. Rather than playing video games late into the night, he plays video games when he wakes up in the morning before he goes to class. He was also taught some relaxation techniques, including deep breathing and guided imagery.

He stated that his neurologist made some changes in his medications and that, in addition to maintaining a routine sleep-and-wake schedule, which he feels has been beneficial, the change in medication has also been positive. He has been working with his social worker to try to find part-time employment and applied for a part-time hospital position. He was hired at a local hospital working as an administrative assistant, and the hospital offers transportation via a shuttle bus for their employees so he does not have to focus on transportation issues.

He stated that therapy has helped him to not feel as limited as he thought he was. He also stated that while his twenties may be difficult because his friends will be staying out late, "I only have to deal with it for ten more years, and then people start to settle down and keep better sleep regiments—they will be just like me."

Case Study: Narcolepsy Type 1

Adrina is a 32-year-old female who is employed as a chef and was diagnosed with narcolepsy type 1 approximately one month ago at an out-of-state sleep center. Adrina stated that she had been falling asleep frequently within the last year but sought treatment after she fell asleep without warning at work while cutting meat off the bone in the midafternoon. She was rushed to the emergency room because she had significantly lacerated her left hand and required 55 stitches. The emergency room physician gave her pain and numbing medication before the stitches; however, at one point during the stitching procedure, Adrina collapsed without warning. The physician became concerned with the reason for the emergency room visit and the current cataplexy episode. He conducted a full medical history and focused on the symptoms of narcolepsy. Based on her responses, the physician referred her to a sleep center for evaluation.

Results of her MSL, Epworth Sleepiness Scale, and overnight sleep polysomnogram resulted in a diagnosis with narcolepsy type 1. She was prescribed an antidepressant for treatment of her narcolepsy symptoms. Within two weeks, she stated that she was more tired in the day and had an increase in sleep episodes while working. At this time, she was offered a sous chef position at a top restaurant in Portland, Oregon, so she moved from San Diego to Portland. However, she was still reporting falling asleep while preparing food and cooking. She stated that her most recent injury occurred when she fell asleep while cooking and received second-degree burns. She presents today for reevaluation.

Her neurologist added a Modafinil (amphetamine) prescription because her narcolepsy symptoms were severe. The neurologist did not change dosage or timing of her antidepressant medication. Within one week, Adrina was no longer falling asleep while at work cooking and preparing food. She now takes a 20-minute nap at the same time every day (1:00–1:20 p.m.). She provided her employer with a physician's letter to show a medical need for a short nap, and her employer has been exceedingly supportive.

Adrina was also educated about positive sleep-hygiene behaviors. She was instructed to keep a sleep diary and educated on the following: maintaining consistent sleep and wake times, having a comfortable sleep environment, limiting evening caffeine intake, avoiding heavy meals (high in carbohydrates) before bedtime, and so on. She was also educated on the importance of limiting strong emotional stimuli that can cause cataplexic attacks and to inform family, friends, and coworkers of the need to tone down jokes to control laugher or other strong emotional stimuli, such as crying.

Two weeks later, Adrina returned for her follow-up appointment. She continued to report no work-related accidents or injuries and has continued to take daytime naps. She uses her break to lie down. She stated that she feels alert and energized throughout the day but begins to feel sleepy during the early evening. Her neurologist added a short-acting methylphenidate to assist with alertness during the early to late evening. Review of her sleep diary demonstrated that she is engaging in sleep-promoting behaviors and keeping consistent sleep and wake routines. She stated that she does not drink alcohol but enjoys drinking tea and has eliminated caffeinated tea beverages before bedtime. She has switched to decaffeinated hot tea before bedtime and finds it relaxing and sleep promoting.

Adrina returned for her follow-up appointment, and the addition of the methylphenidate medication proved to be efficacious. She is able to work without sleepiness episodes and denies any sleep related accidents or injuries. Adrina stated that the key to powering through the afternoon at work is her power nap. No issues were noted with her sleep diary upon review.

Adrina was followed up for two years for minimal changes in medication adjustments. Overall, she did not have another work injury or accident and enjoyed her work. She became engaged one year ago and moved out of state prior to getting married, and so contact with her was lost.

Case Study

Amy is a 39-year-old mother of two children (one adult and one 9-year old) who is employed at a major pharmaceutical company in the research and development area. She was referred to the sleep clinic because she fell asleep while driving and was in an automobile accident. She was rushed to the emergency room and admitted to the hospital. Testing ruled out a seizure disorder or other medical disorders. She underwent a PSG and MSLT and was diagnosed with narcolepsy type 2. No instances of obstructive sleep apnea, leg movement disorder, and so on, were observed. She denies a history of cataplexic events but, for the last two years, has fallen asleep while talking, eating, and working and admits to having sleep paralysis episodes. She denies having any work-related injuries or accidents. She was asked not to drive an automobile until further notice.

Amy was prescribed Modafinil to improve daytime alertness and to reduce the episodes of falling asleep unintentionally. She was educated on sleep-hygiene behaviors and given a sleep diary. She was asked to follow up in two weeks but was instructed to call her neurologist to see if medication adjustments needed to be made prior to her follow-up call.

Amy presented for her appointment and stated that the Modafinil improved her daytime sleepiness, but she still experienced some daytime sleepiness. She also stated that she had two sleep attacks while working during the day since her last visit. She again denied any accident or injuries—she just missed attending a team meeting. Her sleep diary revealed that she eats dinner several hours before bedtime and has light meals. She does not exercise in the late evening but walks her dog for approximately 20 minutes upon arriving home at five o'clock. She denied drinking or smoking—not even socially. Her last cup of caffeinated coffee is at eleven in the morning. She stated that she uses her lunch break at noon to take a power nap. She goes to her car and sets her mobile alarm clock for a 20-minute nap, and then returns to work to finish out her lunch hour. Last, her neurologist adjusted her medication, and she was asked to return in two weeks.

Amy stated that the change in her Modafinil dosage significantly improved her daytime sleepiness, and she denies having any "unwanted sleep" episodes. She feels more alert during the day and has not missed a meeting. She still is not driving. Review of her sleep diary showed that she was sleeping well and throughout the night and woke up feeling refreshed. There were no sleep behaviors of concern or issue to address during the session.

Amy continues to be followed, and her narcolepsy is controlled with Modafinil. She received a medical release to drive an automobile; she has not wanted to drive an automobile because she is concerned about "uncontrollable sleep" while at the wheel. She was recently promoted and enjoys her work life. Other than driving, she is living a full life and reports good to excellent quality-of-life ratings across all levels and domains.

References

American Academy of Sleep Medicine (2014). *International classification of sleep disorders* (3rd ed.). Darien, IL: American Academy of Sleep Medicine.

A. Bahammam (2007). Periodic leg movements in narcolepsy patients: Impact on sleep architecture. *ACTA Neurological Scandinavia, 115*, 351–355. https://doi.org/10.1111/j.160-0404.2006.000754

P. F. Bladin (2000). Narcolepsy—Cataplexy and psychoanalytic theory of sleep and dreams. *Journal of History of the Neurosciences, 9*(2), 1203–1217.

C. W. Christine, W. J. Marks, & J. L. Ostrem (2012). Development of Parkinson's disease in patents with narcolepsy. *Journal of Neurological Transmission, 119*, 697–699.

H. R. Colten, & B. M. Altevogt (Eds.) (2006). *Sleep disorders and sleep deprivation: An unmet public health problem*. Washington, DC: The National Academies Press.

A. De la Herrán Arita, K. Alberto, A. Equihua-Benítez, & R. Drucker-Colin (2013). Treatment of cataplexy. *Expert Opinion on Orphan Drugs, 1*, 199–210. https://doi.org/10.1517/21678707.2013.765359

P. P. Doghramji, J. A. Lieberman, & M. L. Gordon (2007). Stay awake. Understanding, diagnosing and successfully managing narcolepsy. *The Journal of Family Medicine, 56*(11), 518–532.

L. Dunne, P. Patel, E. L. Maschauer, I. Morrison, & R. L. Riha (2016). Misdiagnosis of narcolepsy. *Sleep Breath, 20,* 1277–1284.

A. Gupta, G. Shulda, V. Goyal, A. Srivastava, & M. Behari (2012). Clinical polysomnographic characteristics of 20 North Indian patients with narcolepsy: A seven-year experience from a neurology service sleep clinic. *Neurology India, 60*(1), 75–78.

Harvard Medical School. *Narcolepsy: Self-Care.* Retrieved November 18, 2019, from http://healthysleep.med.harvard.edu/narcolepsy/treating-narcolepsy/self-care

S. J. Kim, I. K. Lyco, Y. S. Lee, J. U. Lee, S. Joon, J. E. Kim, et al. (2009). Gray matter deficits in young adults with narcolepsy. *ACTA Neurology Scandinavia, 119,* 61–67. https://doi.org/10.1111/j.1600-0404.2008.01063

K. T. Lee, C. S. Lee, & I. Y. Yoon (2015). Different of excessive daytime sleepiness: Survival analysis for remission. *ACTA Neurological Scandinavia, 134,* 35–41. https://doi.org/ 10.1111/anc12504

C. E. Mahoney, A. Cogswell, I. J. Koralnik, & T. E. Scammell (2019). The neurobiological basis of narcolepsy. *Nature Reviews Neuroscience, 20*(2), 83–93.

Mayo Clinic (2019). *Narcolepsy.* Retrieved December 19, 2019, from https://www.mayoclinic.org/diseases-conditions/narcolepsy/symptoms-causes/syc-20375497

Y. Melamed, Y. Delayahu, & D. Paleacu (2009). Narcolepsy and psychotic states—A case report. *Israel Journal Psychiatry Related Sciences, 1,* 70–73.

V. Mysliwiec, & M. S Brock (2018). Time for a standardized clinical assessment for narcolepsy with obstructive sleep apnea. *Sleep Breath, 22,* 49–50. https://doi.org/10.1007/s11325-017-1516-3

S. Nevisimalova, J. Pisko, J. Buskova, D. Kemlink, P. Prihodova, K. Sonka, & J. Skibova (2013). Narcolepsy: Clinical differences and association with other sleep disorders in different age groups. *Journal of Neurology, 260,* 767–775. https://doi.org/10.1001/s00415-012-6702-4

E. Olunu, R. Kimo, E. Olufunmbi Onigbinde, M. A. Uduak Akpanobong, I. E. Enang, M. Osanakpo, et al. (2018). Sleep paralysis, a medical condition with a diverse cultural interpretation. *International Journal of Applied and Basic Medical Research, 8*(3): 137–142.

J. Peacock, & R. M. Benca (2010). Narcolepsy: Clinical features, comorbidities & treatment. *Indian Journal Medical Research, 131,* 338–349.

F. Pizza, S. Tartarott, R. Poryazova, C. R. Bauman, & C. L. Bassetti (2013). Sleep-disordered breathing and periodic limb in narcolepsy with cataplexy: A systematic analysis of 35 consecutive patients. *European Neurology, 70,* 22–26. https://doi.org/10.1159/00 0349819

K. Ramar, & E. J. Olson (2013). Management of common sleep disorders. *American Family Physician, 88*(4), 231–238.

C. Sabanayagam, & A. Shankar (2010). Sleep duration and cardiovascular disease: Results from the Nation Health Interview Survey. *Sleep, 33*(8), 1037–1042.

T. E. Scammell, & C. J. Winrow (2011). Orexin Receptors: Pharmacology and Therapeutic Opportunities. *Annual Review of Pharmacology and Toxicology, 51*, 243–266.

C. Schiappa, S. Scarpelli, A. D'Atri, M. Gorgoni, & L. De Gennaro (2018). Narcolepsy and emotional experience: A review of the literature. *Behavioral and Brain Functions,* 14, 19.

M. Seiminski, K. Chwojnicki, T. Sarkanen, & M. Partinen (2017). The relationship between orexin levels and blood pressure changes in patients with narcolepsy. *PLoS One, 12*(10), e185975. https:// doi.org /10.1341/journal.pone.0185975

K. Suzuki, M. Miyamoto, T. Miyamoto, Y. Inoue, K. Matsui, S. Nishida, et al. (2015). The prevalence and characteristics of primary headache and dream-enacting behavior in Japanese patients with narcolepsy or idiopathic hypersomnia. *PLoS One, 10*(9), e0139229.

S. Taheri, J. M. Zeitzer, & E. Mignot (2002). The role of hypocretins (orexins) in sleep regulation and narcolepsy. *Annual Review Neuroscience, 25,* 283–313. https://doi.org/10.1146/annrev.neuro.25.112701.142826

N. F., Watson, T. G. Ton, T. D. Koepsell, V. H. Gersuk, & W. T. Longstreth, Jr. (2010). Does narcolepsy symptom severity vary according to HLA-DQB1*0602 allele status? *Sleep, 33*(1), 29–35.

CHAPTER 7

Pediatric Sleep

At least 25% of children have a sleep-related problem between infancy and adolescence, and functional consequences due to poor sleep duration or quality are common (Mindell & Owens, 2009). Sleep in the pediatric population is necessary and optimal for health and overall functioning. Sleeping the number of recommended hours on a regular basis is associated with better health outcomes, including improved attention, behavior, learning, memory, emotional regulation, quality of life, and mental and physical health (Paruthi et al., 2016; Sheldon, Ferber, Kryger, & Gozal, 2012).

The American Academy of Pediatrics (AAP) (2016) issued a statement of endorsement supporting the American Academy of Sleep Medicine (AASM) guidelines outlining recommended sleep duration for children from infants to teens (Paruthi et al., 2016).

The 2016 consensus group (consisting of 13 sleep and research experts) recommends the following sleep hours (adapted from AAP, 2016):

- Infants 4–12 months should sleep 12–16 hours per 24 hours (including naps) on a regular basis to promote optimal health.
- Children 1–2 years of age should sleep 11–14 hours per 24 hours (including naps) on a regular basis to promote optimal health.
- Children 3–5 years of age should sleep 10–13 hours per 24 hours (including naps) on a regular basis to promote optimal health.
- Children 6–12 years of age should sleep 9–12 hours per 24 hours on a regular basis to promote optimal health.
- Teenagers 13–18 years of age should sleep 8–10 hours per 24 hours on a regular basis to promote optimal health.

Additionally, the group identified that adequate quantity of sleep (sleep duration) for age on a regular basis leads to improved attention, behavior, learning, memory, emotional regulation, quality of life, and mental and physical health. Conversely, not getting enough sleep each night is associated with an increase in injuries, hypertension, obesity, and depression, especially for teens, who may experience increased risk of self-harm or suicidal thoughts. One can conclude that sleep has its importance in daily functioning, and children need to get the appropriate amount of sleep for optimal functioning. Like adults, children need to have age-appropriate quality and quantity of sleep. Timing of sleep is also an important component of sleep.

Pediatric Sleep-Wake Cycles

Fetal Sleep

Like newborns, fetuses spend most of their time sleeping. At 32 weeks, a fetal baby will sleep between 90 and 95% of the day, which is indistinguishable from newborn sleep (Bilich, 2002). Electroencephalogram (EEG) patterns reveal that some of these hours are spent in deep sleep, some in rapid eye movement (REM) sleep, and some in an indeterminate state (Sheldon et al., 2012). The brain is not entirely developed, so there is a state of indeterminate sleep. REM sleep is similar to adult sleep—movement of eyes during REM sleep (Hopson, 1998). EEG patterns at six months show additional differential. As the infant's brain develops during the first year of life, increasingly complicated patterns of REM and non-REM (NREM) sleep emerge. At this point, sleep is 50% REM and 50% NREM. Scientists further postulate that fetuses may dream during sleep (DiPietro, Costigan, & Voegtline, 2015).

Newborn Sleep (0–3 Months)

Newborns sleep the majority of the 24 hours per day and some 16 hours on an average, and the sleep-wake cycle interacts with the need to be changed, fed, and taken care of. The total amount of newborn sleep is approximately 10–18 hours per day, with 5 or fewer hours spent awake (Kryger, Roth, & Dement, 2011). The sleep period varies in length from a few minutes to several hours, during which newborns are often active, twitching their arms and legs, smiling, sucking, and generally appearing restless (Nationwide Children's Hospital, 2019). During sleep, it is normal for newborns and babies to have pauses of 15–20 seconds between breaths. As the child matures, these pauses become less frequent and shorter.

Newborns express their need to sleep in different ways. For instance, some newborns will rub their eyes, cry, and fuss, trying to express the need for sleep. Implementing good sleep hygiene is important—putting babies to bed when they are sleepy. It is essential for newborns to learn to associate their beds with sleep (just like adult sleep-hygiene behaviors). Exposure to bright light, daytime play, and environmental noise will keep newborns less likely to sleep during the day (Nationwide Children's Hospital, 2019).

Infant Sleep (4–12 Months)

By six to nine months of age, nocturnal feedings are less likely to occur because infants are generally sleeping through the night (Sleep Foundation, 2020). Daytime naps are needed during infancy and toddler years. Infants typically sleep 9–12 hours during the night and take 30-minute to two-hour naps, one to four times a day—fewer as they reach the age of one. Parents need to keep practicing adaptive sleep-hygiene behaviors to avoid separation anxiety and to help infants feel comfortable falling asleep in their cribs or beds without the need to be held. Infants are also more likely to sleep through the night if they can soothe themselves back to sleep if they awaken.

Toddler Sleep (1–2 Years)

Toddlers sleep increases to 11–14 hours of sleep compared to newborn sleep (Kryger et al., 2011; Sleep Foundation, 2020). At approximately 1.5 years of age, naptimes decrease from two naps to one nap per day. The nap time will be between one and three hours. Parents need to be cognizant of the time of naps because naps close to a toddler's bedtime may interfere with sleep onset. By the age of two years, most toddlers have spent more time asleep than awake. Overall, a child will spend 40% of his or her childhood asleep (Sleep Foundation, 2020). Toddlers also tend to gravitate toward transition objects. A particular toy, blanket, or pacifier takes on a level of comfort or stability for them as they learn to personally regulate themselves (Davis, Parker, & Montgomery, 2004; Markt & Johnson, 1993). The object is termed "transitional" because it not only is used both day and night but also represents safety. Many hospitals, police officers, and so on, will give a blanket, toy, or doll to a child as a signifier of safety and comfort that is most often associated with the maternal figure (i.e., mother).

Toddlers tend to be more active than adults during the night (e.g., movement in sleep). This age group may also have difficulties initiating sleep, and sleep-maintenance issues are common. They are more likely to get out of bed. For example, some toddlers have been found wandering in the home and even playing with their toys while their parents were asleep in the middle of the night.

Preschoolers Sleep (3–5 Years)

Preschoolers typically sleep 11–13 hours each night (very similar to toddler sleep), and after age five, naps may be reduced to one or no naps. Similar to toddlers, preschoolers also have issues with falling and staying asleep during the night. With further development of imagination, preschoolers commonly experience nighttime fears and nightmares. In addition, sleepwalking and sleep terrors peak during preschool years (Nationwide Children's Hospital, 2019; Sheldon et al., 2012; Sleep Foundation, 2020).

School-Age Children Sleep (6–13 Years)

In children aged 6–12 years old, total sleep time varies between 8 and 10 hours. Sleep patterns also change in terms of a reduction in deep sleep (also called delta sleep). The amount of time until sleep cycles to REM sleep is reduced from 140 minutes to 125 minutes. The transitional objects of toddlerhood continue to be utilized in this period, but as children gain more autonomy and empowerment, they are less likely to have a transitional object after the age of 13 years.

As children continue to mature in this school-age population, they are more active from a social and physical perspective and tend to take on more responsibility and ownership of things. For instance, homework tends to be more demanding, social functioning with friends and family increases, and sports and hobbies tend be of greater interest than in earlier years and come to dominate adolescents' schedules. Interest in hobbies, texting and talking on the phone, reading, watching television, and surfing the internet can negatively impact sleep. This may lead to sleep-onset delays because the children stay up past their bedtimes to keep engaging in these activities, or these activities tend to be mentally stimulating and delay sleep onset. The consequence of this is a reduction in sleep and accruing sleep deprivation. Parents and teachers may notice a decline in school performance.

In adolescence, the sleep-efficiency gains made in childhood are tested. The total sleep time need of eight to nine hours is stable in adolescence; however, the adolescent behaviors intrude upon this. Preferences for social activities (e.g., social media, peer activities, sports) begin to dominate many adolescents' schedules. The consequence of this is a reduction in sleep and accruing sleep deprivation. Carskadon's (2011) research established the advancement of the adolescent's readiness for sleep. Her empirical data clearly identified an adolescent median bedtime of 11:30–11:45—some 90 minutes later than the childhood bedtime of 10:00 p.m. that is generally established in many Western households.

Pediatric Sleep Disorders

The pediatric population experience the same classification of sleep disorders as adult. The presentation of the sleep disorder may be different. For instance, symptoms of obstructing sleep apnea are vastly different in children than in adults. The most common sleep disorders experienced by children are the following (Sheldon et al., 2012):

- Arousal disorders
- Snoring
- Upper airway resistance syndrome (UARS)
- Obstructive sleep apnea (OSA)
- Central sleep apnea (CSA)
- Restless legs syndrome
- Insomnia
- Nighttime sleep behaviors/parasomnias

Sleep disorders in infants, children, and adolescents are common. Studies have shown that poor sleep quality or quantity in children are associated with a host of problems, including academic, behavioral, developmental, and social difficulties; weight abnormalities; and other health problems (Stanford Health Care, 2019). While pediatric sleep problems affect the child, the sleep problems can be more widespread, impacting family dynamics and parental or sibling sleep. The most common sleep disorders identified by Sheldon et al. (2012) not only affect the timing and duration sleep but also cause physiological problems, such as obstructive sleep apnea; abnormal or disruptive behaviors during sleep, such as sleepwalking (or other parasomnias symptoms) that occur near sleep onset, including restless legs syndrome; and daytime symptoms, such as excessive sleepiness, cataplexy, and others (Paruthi et al., 2016; Stanford Health Care, 2019). Furthermore, these researchers state that while children may suffer from the same sleep problems as adults, the cause and presentation of symptoms may be very different. Last, children can develop insomnia disorders, and adolescents can develop delayed sleep-phase syndrome (sleep is delayed by two hours or more from conventional bedtimes), and these findings can be related to child development (Carskadon, 2011).

Obstructive sleep apnea in childhood is a serious concern. Approximately, 3–12% of children snore, compared to obstructive sleep apnea syndrome, which affects 1–10% of children (Chan, Edman, & Koltai, 2004). Most of these children have mild symptoms, and many outgrow the condition. In the developing child, pharynx and tonsil growth may prevent a patent airway (Zastrow, Grando, de Carvalho, da Silva Rath, & Calvo, 2007), leading to breathing difficulties, especially while sleeping. To be diagnosed with sleep apnea, children are generally administered the same procedures as adults (e.g., nocturnal polysomnogram). General treatment may include surgical intervention, continuous positive airway pressure (CPAP), or an oral appliance. However, CPAP is only effective in 20% of children because children grow rapidly, frequent follow-up visits are necessary, and the mask must be adjusted at least every six months (Chan et al., 2004). Referral to a surgeon, ENT, and orthodontist may be recommended. In some instances, genetics may play a factor in the malformation of the face and oropharynx, leading children to a disposition for sleep apnea. Last, if the child is obese, weight reduction can be an effective treatment for obstructive sleep apnea.

Consequences of untreated obstructive sleep apnea include failure to thrive, enuresis, irritability, excessive daytime sleepiness, attention-deficit disorder, behavior problems, poor academic performance, and cardiopulmonary disease (Chan et al., 2004). These researchers also concluded that children five years and older commonly exhibit enuresis (bed-wetting), behavior problems, deficient attention span, and failure to thrive, in addition to snoring.

Children's behavior related to sleep involves, at times, their reluctance to go to sleep. A special issue of *Time* Magazine (2019) highlights the topic of sleep. *Time* reported that "adequate sleep duration for age on a regular basis leads to improved attention, behavior, learning, memory, emotional regulation, quality of life, and mental and physical health." Not getting enough sleep each night is associated with an increase in injuries, hypertension, obesity, and depression, especially for teens who may experience increased risk of self-harm or suicidal thoughts (AAP, 2016).

Treatment

Cognitive and Behavior Modification

Sleep hygiene is the most common behavior modification treatment that is used to address pediatric sleep disorders/disturbances. Additionally, there are cognitive and behavioral techniques used to modify sleep behavior, and these include sleep-restriction therapy, stimulus control, cognitive therapy, and relaxation training. The Sleep Foundation (2020) states that many toddlers experience sleep problems, including resisting going to bed and nighttime awakenings. Implementing adaptive sleep-hygiene principles generally alleviates the disturbed sleep because consistent bedtime and wake times are scheduled. Nighttime fears and nightmares are also common and, unless they occur frequently causing impairment and distress, will generally dissipate with time. However, daytime sleepiness or significant alertness and energy can also be problematic and are reasons to seek consultation with a sleep clinician. Sleep deprivation (inadequate sleep) and disturbed sleep can negatively influence overall emotional function and lead to emotional and behavioral problems. Of concern would be attention deficit hyperactive disorder (ADHD) and cognitive issues that would affect learning.

Behavior modification treatment generally includes the child and parent(s). This type of treatment uses scheduled awakenings, positive reinforcement, and other techniques (e.g., sleep hygiene) and may be helpful in some cases of sleep disorders (Stanford Health Care, 2019).

Cognitive Behavioral Therapy

Childhood and adolescent insomnia diagnoses are more common than most people realize. The cognitive behavioral intervention for insomnia has been adapted to address sleep problems in children. Dewald-Kaufmann, de Bruin, and Michael (2019) used a combination of cognitive behavioral therapy for insomnia (CBT-i) techniques in treating pediatric (school-aged children and adolescents) insomnia. These techniques included bedtime shifts (including sleep restriction), stimulus control therapy, sleep hygiene techniques, thought challenging, psychoeducation, and relaxation techniques. They also integrated the parents with the insomnia treatment. The integration of parents, especially in school-aged children with insomnia, is highly recommended. While the study sample size was small, the results were promising.

There are pediatric insomnia questionnaires in addition to the CBT-i, such as the University of Chicago pediatric insomnia questionnaire, created to assist cognitive behavior therapists in treating the insomniac pediatric population. How children endorse the questionnaire will assist CBT-i therapists in creating treatment goals for healthy sleep. Generally, intervention focuses on parent training that facilitates the scheduling of consistent bedtimes and the development of presleep rituals for easing the transition to sleep and engaging the child to adapt to healthy sleep hygiene.

Sleep Hygiene

The importance of sleep hygiene is no different between adults and children. Children are reluctant to go to bed, and the reluctance is variable. The group (typically 5–8 years) found that adequate sleep duration for age on a regular basis leads to improved attention, behavior, learning, memory, emotional regulation, quality of life, and mental and physical health. Not getting enough sleep each night is associated with an increase in injuries, hypertension, obesity, and depression, especially for teens who may experience increased risk of self-harm or suicidal thoughts (AAP, 2016). Most sleep clinicians do not recommend that children or adolescents have televisions in their bedrooms. Children should have similar presleep, calming behaviors as adults, such as turning off television, computers, internet, and cellular phones (no texting or talking) and not participating in other behaviors that are mentally stimulating. For instance, if a child enjoys reading, this is a mentally stimulating activities and it is doubtful that he or she will want to stop reading at the desired bedtime if the chapter is of interest. Establishing scheduled sleep and wake times starting with infancy and through adolescence is critical for children to get the appropriate amounts of sleep for their age group (AAP, 2016). Parents and caregivers are also encouraged to assist children in getting adequate sleep. When children visit their grandparents, the grandparents may sometimes keep the children up past their bedtimes because they are enjoying their company. It is important to keep sleep schedules consistent. Last, the bedroom should be a calming, quiet environment that avoids light (e.g., adding blackout curtains) and where the temperature is consistent with being able to fall asleep.

Last, younger children tend to want to sleep with their parents (i.e., cosleeping and bed sharing). The reader is cautioned that safe sleep practices and habits are essential for keeping children (especially infants) safe. The potential for the sleeper to roll over on an infant while bed sharing or cosleeping and suffocate the infant is of great concern. Safety is the primary concern for why infants should sleep in their own beds. Infants should always be placed on their backs when lying in bed. Older children who sleep in their parents' beds may not want to leave the comfort and security of sleeping with parents as they get older. This habit can be hard to break in many children because they do not understand why they are being asked to sleep in their own beds. It may be beneficial to avoid cosleeping with parents so that they can learn to feel safe and secure sleeping in their own beds.

Medication Management

While behavior modification treatment may address some sleep issues, some childhood sleep disorders may require medication management. A sleep clinician can recommend medications or supplements to treat a specific sleep disorder or underlying condition. The most common contributors of sleeplessness in children, including medical sleep disorders that lead to disturbed sleep, include but are not limited to sleep-disordered breathing (SDB), restless legs syndrome (RLS), and periodic limb movement disorder (PLMD); circadian rhythm disorders, such as delayed sleep phase syndrome (DSPS); and problems in child-parent behaviors, such as behavioral insomnia of childhood (BIC), sleep-onset association (SOA), or limit-setting (LS) type (Mindell & Owens, 2009). Treatment can include prescription and over-the-counter medications.

Effects and Costs

In Society

Poor sleep hygiene places the child at risk for the development of sleep disorders and poor health conditions. Mental awareness and school performance are just some of the areas in which deficits may appear. If children are tired or sleepy during the day or have poor academic performance, other children may make fun of them and they may feel like outcasts.

In Relationships

Children with poor sleep are more likely to become involved in sedentary activities. The low expenditure of energy to sit and watch television all day is preferred over sports activities, for example. They may reduce social interactions, preferring to sleep than spend time with friends.

Case Study: Childhood Obstructive Sleep Apnea

Davie was a 13-year-old male, the youngest of three children, and was accompanied by both his parents. Davie was below average in height compared to his peers and was significantly above average in weight for his age. Davie's parents brought him to the sleep clinic for an evaluation due to poor academic performance, irritability, and loud snoring. He occasionally wet the bed and would not let his parents know because he was ashamed. He was also recently in a couple of school fights because he stated that he was being picked on by school bullies, who called him "slow, fat, and stupid." His neck was 16 inches in circumference. He was unable to stay awake while in school, driving as a passenger in a car, at the movie theater, studying, and watching television. He refused to play outdoors with his siblings because he stated that he had no energy. During a recent physical education class, he had to run up and down the basketball court. He was very tired that day and tripped when running and sprained his ankle. Additionally, he was feeling sleepy while riding his bike from a friend's home and was not paying attention. He hit the curb and fell over the handlebars, with no major injuries.

Davie denied complaints of nocturnal leg movements, difficulty falling and staying asleep, or having any REM or NREM sleep issues. He stated that he generally went to bed at 9:30 p.m. and woke up during the night "gasping for air." He described "gasping for air" as a frightening experience because he was afraid he would not wake up and would suffocate. He also stated that when he woke up, he still felt sleepy. Without his parents or siblings forcing him to get up, he would stay in bed and not get up for hours later. His parents also noted that it looked like he had cessation of breathing during the night. He also snored in any position, and his siblings often complained that they could hear the snoring across the house. He was generally the last to be ready for any occasion when the family had to leave for an engagement. His mother stated that she got very frustrated and embarrassed because Davie would fall asleep and start to snore loudly during Sunday mass.

Results of his Epworth Sleep Score reveal that he was significantly sleepy during the day. He was scheduled for a nocturnal polysomnogram (PSG). His PSG results showed that he had significant OSA with loud snoring, and CPAP treatment and surgical consultation for removal of his tonsils was discussed with Davie and his parents at their next follow-up appointment. His parents stated that they had been educating themselves about treating children with CPAP, and they would like to try it. When Davie was asked what he wanted to do, he stated that he did not want to get his tonsils removed. He stated that he would be willing to try anything, as long as it made him feel better and helped to stop the bullying.

Davie was educated about CPAP and was fitted with a face mask. He stated that he thought it was "cool" because he felt like Darth Vader from *Star Wars*. He and his parents were educated regarding healthy sleep hygiene behaviors as part of his treatment plan. Last, weight loss and the relationship to obstructive sleep apnea were discussed. Davie stated, "I know that I am fat and lazy, but I do not want to be that way. I want to be like other kids who get to do fun things." His mother stated that she was going to schedule an appointment with a nutritionist.

When Davie returned for his follow-up and compliance visit, he was 99% compliant and stated that he felt better and had more energy. He described sitting in class was easier than before because he did not have to "fight to stay awake." His mother stated that he had been doing slightly better in school.

Additionally, she took Davie to a nutritionist who asked him to keep a food log and had been educating Davie and his mother about appropriate portion sizes, different food groups, and the importance of adding snacks to his diet. Davie was also told to avoid eating heavy meals toward bedtime hours. He was also advised not to drink soda or too much fruit juice due to the sugar content. Davie's mother was choosing healthier meal options instead of letting him eat fast food meals that are high in carbohydrates.

His one-month appointment revealed that he was 100% compliant and had lost six pounds. He continued to feel more energy during the day and woke up feeling more refreshed. He was spending more time with his siblings, playing with them outdoors, than he was previously. He also was not falling asleep when playing video games or watching movies.

His two-month appointment revealed that he was 98% compliant (he was recently sick and missed a day or two of using his CPAP because he was up during the night due to a stomach flu). His mother reported that he lost an additional nine pounds, and his clothes no longer fit him. He volunteered to do extra chores to earn more money to save up for something. He continued to improve at school, and his teacher stated that he while he was quiet, he was attentive during the day. He would ask a question if he did not understand something.

At Davie's three-month appointment, he was refitted for a face mask because he stated that air was coming out of it and bothering him. His compliance was 99%, and he stated that he lost another six pounds. He and his father now took the dog for a two-mile walk. He continued to be alert at school, and his grades were improving. His parents said that he was no longer irritable or moody, and his temperament was more loving and calmer. He was following his nutritional counseling, and his mother was slowly introducing him different, healthier foods.

At his four-month appointment, compliance was 100%. Davie stated that he was invited to a sleepover at his friend's house, but he was afraid to go because he did not want his friend to make fun of his CPAP machine, and if he did not bring the machine, he would snore. Davie and his mother discussed going to the party and weighed the pros and cons of going with the CPAP machine versus not bringing it. Davie lost an additional three pounds.

Davie's five-month appointment revealed 100% CPAP compliance, and he earned his first A on a school test. He continued to be more active and was interested in learning how to play tennis. Davie stated that he did not spend the night at his friend's house. His mother picked him up at 10:00 p.m., and he returned the next morning to spend the rest of the day with his friends. He stated that his friend was disappointed but happy to know that he would return in the morning. Davie happily reported that he lost another four pounds and was swimming at the gym with his father after they took the dog for a walk.

Davie's six-month appointment revealed that he remained at 100% CPAP compliance. His mother stated that he no longer snored loudly. She described returning home from a long day at her sister's home, and all the children fell asleep on the return trip, and Davie did not snore. He lost a total of 28 pounds. He no longer fit in the new clothes his mother recently purchased for him. Davie's mood and affect were notable different from his initial presentation.

Davie was followed for a total of 2.4 years and was no longer using CPAP due to his weight loss. At his last visit, he stated that his goal was to be on the honor roll. He played a variety of sports with his friends and family. He enjoyed running during the early evening with the family dog. He no longer had academic issues and had grown 4.75 inches in the last two years.

References

American Academy of Pediatrics (2016). *American Academy of Pediatrics supports childhood sleep guidelines.* Retrieved December 19, 2019, from https://www.aap.org/en-us/about-the-aap/aap-press-room

/Pages/American-Academy-of-Pediatrics-Supports-Childhood-Sleep-Guidelines.aspx

M. A. Carskadon (2011). Sleep in adolescents: The perfect storm. *Pediatric Clinics of North America, 58*(3), 637–647. https://doi.org/10.1016/j.pcl.2011.03.003

J. Chan, J. Edman, & P. Koltai (2004). Obstructive sleep apnea in children. *American Family Physician, 69*(5), 1147–1155.

K. A. Bilich (2002). Baby's alertness in the womb. *Parents.* Retrieved November 26, 2019, from, https://www.parents.com/pregnancy/stages/fetal-development/babys-alertness-in-the-womb/

K. F. Davis, K. P. Parker, & G. L. Montgomery (2004). Sleep in infants and young children: Part one: Normal sleep. *Journal of Pediatric Health Care, 18*(2), 65–71.

J. Dewald-Kaufmann, E. de Bruin, & G. Michael (2019). Cognitive Behavioral Therapy for Insomnia (CBT-i) in school-aged children and adolescents. *Sleep Medicine Clinics, 14*(2), 155–165.

J. A. DiPietro, K. A. Costigan, & K. M. Voegtline (2015). Studies in fetal behavior: Revisited, renewed and reimagined. *Monographs of the Society for Research in Child Development, 80*(3), vii–94. https://doi.org/10.1111/mono.v80.3

P. Ferber (2006). *Solve your child's sleep problems* (2nd ed.). New York: Fireside.

M. E. Frank, N. P. Issa, & M. P Stryker (2001). Sleep enhances plasticity in the developing visual cortex. *Neuron, 30*(1), 33–38.

J. L. Hopson (1998, September–October). Fetal psychology. *Psychology Today.* Retrieved April 21, 2021, from www.psychologytoday.com/us/articles/199809/fetal-psychology

I. Iglowstein, W. G. Jennic, L. Molinari, & R. H. Largo (2002). Sleep duration from infancy to adolescence: Reference values and generational trends. *Pediatrics, 111*(2), 302–307.

M. H. Kryger, T. Roth, & W. C. Dement (2011). *Principles and practice of sleep medicine* (6th ed.). Philadelphia, PA: Saunders/Elsevier.

C. Markt, & M. Johnson (1993). Transitional objects, pre-sleep rituals, and psychopathology. *Child Psychiatry and Human Development, 23*, 161–173. https://doi.org/10.1007/BF00707147

K. G. McGary (2018). *How well did you sleep last night and why getting enough sleep matters.* http://kristinmcgary.com/how-well-did-you-sleep-last-night-and-why-getting-enough-sleep-matters.html

J. Mindell, & J. Owens (2009). *A clinical guide to pediatric sleep: Diagnosis and management of sleep problems in children and adolescents.* Philadelphia, PA: Lippincott Williams and Wilkins.

Nationwide Children's Hospital (2019). *Healthy sleep habits for infants and toddlers*. Retrieved December 18, 2019, from https://www.nationwidechildrens.org/family-resources-education/health-wellness-and-safety-resources/helping-hands/healthy-sleep-habits-for-infants-and-toddlers.

S. Paruthi, L. J. Brooks, C. D'Ambrosio, W. A. Hall, S. Kotagal, R. M. Lloyd, et al. (2016). Recommended amount of sleep for pediatric populations: a consensus statement of the American Academy of Sleep Medicine. *Journal of Clinical Sleep Medicine, 12*(6), 785–786.

S. H. Sheldon, R. Ferber, M. H. Kryger, & D. Gozal (2012). *Principles and practice of pediatric sleep medicine* (2nd ed.). New York: Elsevier Inc.

Sleep Foundation (2020). *Children and sleep*. Retrieved January 2, 2020, from https://www.sleepfoundation.org/articles/children-and-sleep

Stanford Health Care (2019). *Pediatric sleep disorder*. Retrieved November 18, 2019, from, https://stanfordhealthcare.org/medical-conditions/sleep/pediatric-sleep-disorders.html

C. Suwanrath, & T. Suntharasaj (2010). Sleep–wake cycles in normal fetuses. *Archives of Gynecology and Obstetrics, 281*, 449–454. https://doi.org/10.1007/s00404-009-1111-3

Time Magazine (2019). *The science of sleep*. Retrieved April 21, 2021, from https://time.com/collection/guide-to-sleep/

M. D. Zastrow, L. J. Grando, A. P. de Carvalho, I. B. da Silva Rath, & M. C. Calvo (2007). A comparative study of the breathing pattern and amount of nasopharynx obstruction by the pharyngeal tonsil in HIV infected and non-infected children. *Brazilian Journal of Otorhinolaryngology, 73*(5), 583–591.

CHAPTER 8

Student Sleep

Young adult college students are at risk of the development of health problems secondary to lifestyle factors such as unmanaged stress, substance use/abuse, and poor sleep. In the student environment, the wellness or health center is the central source of health information and care. However, a sleep specialist or consultant with training in this area may not be available. The young adult college student is typically sleep deprived as a result of poor choices to ignore sleep needs in favor of social schedules by choice or, commonly, by obligation. Young adult college students may prefer streaming television and films, video games, or socializing to the routine of a regular bed and wake time. In surveys, college students self-report feeling more stressed and identify poor sleep as a contributing factor. In a closer examination of these issues, an irregular sleep pattern was found. Varying bedtimes and wake times erode the sleeper's ability to signal to the brain behaviorally that it is sleep time and wake time (Sexton-Radek, 2003).

Reports in the scientific literature identify the association between irregular sleep patterns and poor cognitive performance on short-term tasks such as classroom behavior projects and homework as well as long-term measures such as test scores and grade point average (Gaultney, 2010; Pilcher & Walters, 1997; Schmidt, Richter, Gendolla, & van der Linden, 2010). Recent studies in this area identify that it is typically students with low grades, high stress, and an alertness style that peaks in the evening as more often engaging in last-minute, all-night study. Nationally, poor sleep is considered a public health concern. In their campus health survey, the American College Health Association identified sleep difficulty as second on the list of factors that affected the student's individual's academic performance.

College students who engage in a single night of total sleep deprivation report higher levels of stress, depression, and sleep problems, than students who did not do so, and students who used this as a method of accomplishing college work would be academically weaker as measured by GPA (Thatcher, 2008). College students in psychology courses at a small, liberal arts university responded to questions regarding their sleep habits, mood, and stress levels, including self-reports of their use of "all-nighters." The students were asked about their reasons for either using or abstaining from "all-nighters." An "all-nighter" was defined as a night on which the student remembered staying up past his or her usual wake time, whenever that might be. The participants completed the Morningness/Eveningness (Owl-Lark) Scale, the Pittsburgh Sleep Quality Index (PSQI), the Beck Depression Inventory (BDI), and the Perceived Stress Measure (PSM). These scales are commonly used in sleep studies. The Morningness/Eveningness Scale provides a score describing whether the person's peak energy level is in the morning (i.e., like a chirping lark in the morning) or a peak in the evening (i.e., like the nighttime hooting owl). The Pittsburgh Sleep Quality Index measures a person's self-reported sleep behaviors, such as bedtime, wake time, number of wake-ups after sleep, and sleeplessness. The Beck Depression Inventory is a standard measure used in the sleep research and psychology fields and asks the participant to self-report whether he or she experiences signs and symptoms of depression. All these measures are psychometrically strong in reliability and validity. Nearly twice as many students reported ever having pulled an all-nighter, 63%, as denied having done so, 37%. Among those who reported ever pulling an all-nighter, the reasons were twice as often academic as social. For first-year students only, the last year of high school was also included in the totals reported. About 40% of first-year students reported never using "all-nighters" during their first year of college; about a third reported one, two, three, or four "all-nighters" per week; the remaining 25% of students reported five or more "all-nighters" during the first year. In addition to describing college student sleep quality, results from an investigation such as this points to the level of judgment in college students, in general, in attempting to manage novel situations that seem overwhelming, such as college exams and assignment deadlines. Further, in the group of college students reporting "all-nighters," scores reflecting "eveningness" tendencies, reported lower GPAs, and self-reported low mood were commonly reported (Thatcher, 2008).

There are several ways to define sleep habits and sleep problems. People of all ages struggle with sleep problems, including poor sleep hygiene, but issues with sleep are a common problem in college populations (Anderson-Fye & Floersch, 2011; Sousa, Souza, Masili, & Macedo, 2013). There are a plethora of factors that contribute to sleep complaints and problems within the college student population. For instance, late-night studying, all-nighters, parties, social obligations, work, and alcohol or drug abuse all likely play a role. How do we work with college students who are focusing on academic success despite sleep issues? Gipson, Chilton, Dickerson, Alred, and Hass (2018) and McCabe, Knight, Teter, and Weschler (2003) suggest that we might be able to use academic success as motivation if sleep researchers can establish a relationship between healthy sleep habits and academic success. College students may be more likely to engage in healthy sleep behaviors, including scheduling consistent wake and bedtimes than other adult populations.

van der Schuur, Baumgartner, Sumter, and Valkenburg (2018) suggest that there is a correlation between alcohol consumption, sleep patterns, and academic performance. These researchers randomly distributed surveys to the student population at a liberal arts college. Their findings suggest that alcohol consumption is a significant predictor for duration of sleep, including differences in duration of sleep and timing of sleep during weekday and weekend bedtimes. Kloss et al. (2016) report replication of these findings. Last, these researchers found sleep patterns to be directly associated with GPA. There is a clear link between alcohol consumption compromising academic performance through the effects of alcohol on sleep (Schmidt et al. 2010).

Dworkin (2005) and Galambos, Lascano, Howard, and Maggs (2011) used the Consideration of Future Consequences Scale (CFC), and they surveyed a random sample of college students between the ages of 18 and 41. The CFC focuses on questions about sleep patterns and future career goals. High CFC scores were associated with those college students who were very conscientious and made smart decisions in order to successfully obtain rewards later in life. Additionally, higher scores were associated with college students who maintained regular sleep schedules, and they also had higher grade point averages. The research findings also suggest that the average amount of sleep students achieve per night is associated with their GPAs. Last, for those students who obtain less than five hours of sleep per night appeared to have lower GPAs.

College students' sleep quality may, less commonly, be disturbed due to a sleep disorder (Breslau, Roth, Rosinthal, & Andreski, 1996). A carefully tracked sleep schedule using a wrist accelerometer called an actigraphy is typically used by a sleep specialist to determine diagnosis of insomnia, delayed sleep phase disorder, and other conditions related to insomnia (i.e., environmental conditions, adjustments reaction) following an intake interview and administration of standard measures. The sleep time is illustrated by the black squares, and blank boxes are wake activities. Actigraphic analyses provide a useful analysis of sleep behavior from the sleeper's natural environment. The diagnosis of insomnia can be in terms of sleep onset or sleep maintenance. The sleeper would need to have consistent sleeplessness for 30 days in order to meet the diagnostic criteria. The delayed sleep phase disorder diagnosis is determined when a sleeper's lifestyle schedule causes a disturbance—a later bedtime—in his or her sleep schedule. As a consequence of this behavior, the sleeper, who still requires at least six hours of core sleep, wakes later than the normal wake time, affecting work or class start times. This sleep behavior becomes repetitive, thereby negatively impacting quality of life, academic achievements, and employment success.

Effects and Costs

In Society

Young adults with reduced sleep quality, a common finding, also demonstrate reduced cognitive ability. Measured changes in working memory in a young adult study of sleep documented the difficulty for the young adult to engage meaningfully in society.

At Work

The work of students is their academic lives. In a study of high school seniors using a sleep habits questionnaire, it was found that using prescribed sleep schedules led to reduced daytime sleepiness and increased total sleep time (Prince, Schauer, & Clifton, 2008).

In Relationships

In a recent study of preschool participants' sleep indicated, over time, a relationship between poor sleep of preschoolers and adolescents. The researchers reported the reductions in executive control from poor sleep in the preschoolers sets up a vulnerability to regulations (i.e., poor inhibitory control, poor flexibility/shifting, and low capacity working memory).

Case Study: The Sleep-Deprived Residence Hall Worker

Barb was a junior at a large university, majoring in history and political science. She was in the second month of her employment as a corridor advisor for the third floor of a residence hall that housed 60 student residents. She completed a two-week training course in the summer. She was glad for the position as it afforded her free room and board and a small monthly stipend. Barb began her position this academic term as vice president of the Student Government Association; she aspired to run for president in her senior year. Barb learned a lot with her position in two short months. Her sleep schedule of an 11:30 p.m. bedtime and 6:30 a.m. wake time has been disturbed nightly in the last two months. She had to mediate roommate arguments; disturbances; student calls about room lockouts; and parent/student calls about loud music, too hot or too cold room temperatures, and requests for assistance to extricate a roommate's friend who was staying overnight in the room. Barb valued her job and saw the immediate and long-term value of the learning experiences and opportunities for leadership, but was reevaluating her predicament as she was feeling the effects of her fragmented sleep. Her fitness watch indicated that she slept for 2 hours and 17 minutes, on average, for the last few days; if she took out the weekend nights, which had more extreme disturbances, her average sleep was 2 hours and 42 minutes. Barb had not experienced a drop in her grades but noticed difficulty with attention and concentration, both during classes and as she studied in the library. Barb's health was good. She began her day with a run on the university's outdoor track, one block from the residence hall. Barb had difficulty maintaining her eating and free time schedules as well. She had residence hall training meetings and scheduled meetings with residents that she set to mediate circumstances. Since this blocked her time allotment to go to lunch at the café, she was eating candy bars or skipping breakfast or lunch all together. Lately, she tried to take away fruit and granola bars from one of the meals in the day so she could make healthier "to-go" meals for herself. In the last two days, she had to reduce her running time in order to get to one of the many meetings she scheduled per the protocol of her position to mediate the conflicts and complaints brought to her. Today, while sitting in her reserved study carrel at the library, she found herself falling asleep rather than studying. This event prompted her to make an appointment at the wellness center to address her sleep situation.

Based on this presentation, the sleep specialist consultant at the wellness center explained to Barb that her environment-induced sleep maintenance Insomnia could be best addressed with cognitive behavior treatment (CBT). Barb provided the Excel file of her fitness watch recordings of her sleep. The sleep specialist supported Barb's efforts to maintain her early morning run and commitment to two meals a day and her fruit and granola bar "take away" for a third small meal. A food diary review indicated that Barb consumed one cup of coffee with breakfast per day. While Barb was not overweight, the sleep specialist suggested she eat more protein for her first meal of the day rather than the carbohydrate and sugar items of French toast or pancakes she typically selected. Adding more water, fruits, and fiber, particularly early in the day, was also recommended. Barb was taught to use mindfulness techniques to unwind and, with more advanced work, to use as a means of increasing her focus. Barb was encouraged to try to get some natural sunlight in the early afternoon. She was provided with information about "power naps" and found satisfaction in taking one or two power naps of about 20 minutes each week. In discussion of cognitive variables, Barb was encouraged to speak to her supervisor about techniques to increase her efficacy and reduce the time consumption of so many meetings. Barb related that her supervisor was very helpful in recommending she combine an online warning and consequences system. Barb's discussions inspired the supervisor to use part of the training meetings for the residence advisors to discuss their situations and share strategies to manage the circumstances. Barb learned so much about the basics of sleep that she did her next three monthly programs to the residents on good sleep health topics. Barb felt her six sessions with the sleep specialist consultant were worthwhile, and at the six-month follow-up, she reported being able to return to her 11:30 p.m.–6:30 a.m. sleep schedule and no reductions in her grades.

References

E. P. Anderson-Fye, & J. Floersch (2011). I'm not your typical homework stresses me out kind of girl": Psychological anthropology in research on college student usage of psychiatric medication and mental health services. *Journal of Society for Psychological Anthropology,* 39(4), 501–521.

N. Breslau, T. Roth, L. Rosinthal, & P. Andreski (1996). Sleep disturbances and psychiatric disorders: A longitudinal epidemiological study of young adults. *Biological Psychiatry,* 39, 411–418.

J. Dworkin (2005). Risk taking as developmentally appropriate experimentation for college students. *Journal of Adolescent Research,* 20, 219–241.

N. L. Galambos, D.T. Lascano, A. L. Howard, & J. L. Maggs (2011). Who sleeps best? Longitudinal and covariates of change in sleep quantity, quality and timing across four university years. *Behavioral Sleep Medicine, 11,* 8–22. https://doi.org/10.1080/15402002.2011.598234

J. F. Gaultney (2010). The prevalence of sleep disorders in college students: Impact on academic performance. *Journal of American College Health, 59*(2), 91–97.

C. S. Gipson, J. M. Chilton, S. S. Dickerson, D. Alfred, & B. K. Hass (2018). Effect of a sleep hygiene text message intervention on sleep in college students. *Journal of American College Health, 67*(1), 32–41.

J. D. Kloss, C. O. Nash, C. M. Walsh, E. Culnan, S. Horsey, & K. Sexton-Radek (2016). A "Sleep 101" program for college students improves sleep hygiene knowledge and reduces maladaptive beliefs about sleep. *Behavioral Medicine, 42,* 18–56. https://doi.org/10.1080/08964289.2014.969186

S. E. McCabe, J. R. Knight, C. J. Teter, & H. Weschler (2003). Nonmedical use of prescription stimulants among U.S. college students: Prevalence and correlates from a national survey. *Addiction, 99,* 96–106.

J. J. Pilcher, & A. S. Walters (1997). How sleep deprivation affects psychological variables related to college students' cognitive performance. *College Health, 46,* 121–126.

E. Prince, A. Schauer, & M. Clifton (2008). Evaluating sleep hygiene: Empowering teens to take charge. *Journal of Adolescent Health, 44*(2). https://doi.org/10.1016/j.jadohealth.2008.10.069

R. E. Schmidt, M. Richter, G. H. Gendolla, & M. van der Linden (2010). Young poor sleepers mobilize extra effort in an easy memory task: Evidence from cardiovascular measures. *Journal of Sleep Research, 19,* 487–498.

K. Sexton-Radek (2003). *Sleep quality in young adults.* New York: Mellen Press.

I. C. Sousa, J. C. Souza, F. Massilli, & C. V. Macedo (2013). Changes in sleep habits and knowledge after an educational sleep program in 12th grade students. *Sleep and Biological Rhythms, 11,* 144–153.

P. Thatcher (2008). University students and the all-nighter: Correlates and patterns of students' engagement in a single night of total sleep deprivation. *Behavioral Sleep Medicine, 6,* 16–31.

W. A. van der Schuur, S. E. Baumgartner, S.R. Sumter, & P. M. Valkenburg (2018). Media multitasking and sleep problems: A longitudinal study among adolescents. *Computers in Human Behavior, 81,* 316–324.

CHAPTER 9

Oncology and Sleep

We live our lives, not planning to become ill or be diagnosed with a potentially life-threatening condition. We generally take our health for granted, and we do not focus on "if or when I become ill." Without having any mental preparation or any coping strategies for illness, when we are diagnosed with an illness or disease (acute, chronic, or life threatening), we often do not know how to cope adaptively to the situation. Emotions such as fear and anxiety can interfere with sleep (both quality and quantity). Physicians or medical specialists rarely inquire about how illness, medications, and emotions affect sleep. Treatment generally focuses on addressing the disease, and sleep and other quality of life factors are not addressed.

Medical illness or disease can affect all aspects of sleep: timing, duration, and quality. Sleep can be disrupted by the diagnosis, psychological factors related to coping with an illness, the disease itself, and treatment medications. This chapter will focus on the effects of cancer on sleep. How do people cope with receiving the diagnosis of a potentially life-threatening illness? Instead of sleeping, patients may spend hours at night contemplating how the illness might impact their family and loved ones, relationships, finances, quality of life, work performance, and so on. These thoughts can weigh heavily on someone and interrupt sleep; the interruption can be delayed sleep onset, difficulty returning to sleep, or early morning awakenings. A person may also want to stay in bed and sleep (which could be due to a psychological component, such as depression, or the side effects of treatment or the disease). While this chapter focuses on cancer and sleep, other medical disorders can impact sleep quality and quantity in much the same manner.

Insomnia is a heterogeneous condition that can be symptomatic of an underlying emotional, medical, or substance disorder (Morin, 2000). It can also be an independent disorder with no known etiology, or so-called primary insomnia. Insomnia is the most common sleep disorder reported by cancer patients (Passik, Whitcomb, Kirsh, & Theobald, 2003). It is estimated to affect 30–60% of cancer patients and is highest in females with breast cancer (Savard, Ivers, Savard, & Morin, 2016). Oncologists noticed that alterations in sleep patterns are endemic among their patients (Mills & Graci, 2004), yet sleep problems are rarely assessed in medical or clinic appointments (Graci, 2005). Other concerns, such as morbidity and mortality, appear to take precedence (Mills & Graci, 2004). The cause of chronic sleep difficulties is multifaceted (Graci, 2005; Savard et al., 2015), and there are potential factors associated with the pathogenesis of cancer-related insomnia. The unique contributions of psychologic, medical, treatment side effects, environmental, behavioral, and pharmaceutical pathways on cancer-related insomnia cannot be ignored.

In healthy populations, the incidence of some form of insomnia is about 33%, whereas insomnia severe enough to interfere with daytime functioning is estimated to affect about 10–15% of the general population (Leger et al., 2000; Ohayon, Caulet, Priest, & Guilleminault, 1997; Roth & Ancoli-Israel, 1999). The prevalence, type, and severity of sleep complaints in a cancer population have been difficult to estimate or predict (Fortner, Stepanski, Wang, Kasprowicz, & Durrence, 2002; Savard et al., 2016). Most studies estimate that approximately half of patients with cancer suffer from insomnia, with 23–44% reporting insomnia complaints up to several years following their diagnosis and treatment (Couzi, Helzlsouer, & Fetting, 1995; Lindley, Vasa, Sawyer, & Winer, 1998; Savard, Simard, Blanchet, Ivers, & M. Morin, 2001). It is unknown if the lasting insomnia complaints are due to psychological effects and/or cancer treatment side effects.

Diagnosis and Classification

In a cancer patient population, insomnia complaints are often secondary to underlying psychiatric and medical conditions, and these conditions should be assessed and treated as a first measure (Graci, 2005; Holbrook, Crowther, Lotter, Cheng, & King, 2000a, 2000b; Savard et al., 2016). The *International Classification System of Sleep Disorders* (American Academy of Sleep Medicine, 2001) and the *Diagnostic*

Statistical Manual of Mental Disorders, Fifth Edition (*DSM-5*) (American Psychiatric Association [APA], 2013) are the two classification systems currently used for diagnosing insomnia.

The three main insomnia complaints are difficulty initiating sleep (falling asleep), staying asleep (maintaining sleep), and early morning awakening, and the key feature is that the individual has difficulty initiating and/or returning to sleep. It is essential that clinicians differentiate between patients who are naturally short sleepers (i.e., fewer than six hours) from those whose sleep has been shortened and fragmented from psychologic, medical, pharmaceutical, environmental, and/or behavioral factors (Graci, 2005). The complaint of impaired functioning is a good clue to help distinguish short sleepers from truly disturbed sleepers.

It is important to highlight that a diagnosis of cancer may aggravate an already present insomnia complaint. The two common types of insomnia disorders diagnosed within a cancer population are adjustment and psychophysiological sleep disorders. Adjustment sleep disorder is a condition in which an individual has experienced a significant life stressor (such as the death of a loved one or the diagnosis of a life-threatening illness) that interferes with sleep. This type of sleep disorder is more commonly transient and generally abates within one month (Graci, 2005).

Risk Factors

Insomnia is more common among females, older individuals, and the depressed or anxious (Aldrich, 2000; Graci, 2005; Savard et al., 2016). Additionally, low socioeconomic status, chronic medical illness, low level of education, recent life stressors, and the use of alcohol are also associated with insomnia complaints.

Psychologic Factors

Clinically significant symptoms of depression are present in up to half of cancer patients at some time during their disease course (Ehrenberg, 2000; Massie & Popkin, 1998), yet fewer than 10% of cancer patients are treated with antidepressant medication. Sleep disturbances are indicative in depression. Anxiety is also prevalent in cancer patients, with some significant symptoms occurring in up to 50% of this population (Noyes, Holt, & Massie, 1998; van't Spijker, Trijsburg, & Duivenvoorden, 1997). The diagnosis of cancer as a traumatic event capable of eliciting symptoms of posttraumatic stress disorder has been added to the *DSM-5* (American Psychiatric Association [APA], 2013). This type of anxiety disorder is typically associated with sleep initiation and maintenance difficulties and with vivid nightmares about the traumatic event (Jacobs-Rebhun, Schnurr, & Friedman, 2000).

Medical Factors

The extent of sleep difficulties has been shown to vary with different cancer types (Graci, 2005). Two studies have identified that breast cancer patients treated with radiotherapy had a temporary increase in sleep disturbance (Omne-Pontén, Holmberg, Burns, Adami, & Bergstrom, 1992; Wengstrom, Haggmark, Strander, & Forsberg, 2000). Additionally, prostate cancer patients who are treated with androgen deprivation therapy report an increase in insomnia complaints (Savard et al., 2016).

Davidson, MacLean, Brundage, and Schulze (2002) compared sleep problems in lung cancer patients, breast cancer patients, insomniacs, and healthy controls and found that lung cancer patients had greater decreased sleep efficiency (ratio of time spent sleeping to time spent in bed) compared with breast cancer patients or controls. Silberfarb, Hauri, Oxman, & Schnurr (1993) also reported that lung cancer patients had longer sleep onset latencies, more fragmented sleep, and more stage 1 sleep (light sleep) than breast cancer patients or controls. In another study of sleep and fatigue complaints in a heterogeneous sample of patients, those with lung cancer had the highest prevalence of sleep-related problems (Davidson et al., 2002).

The nighttime sleep disturbance and daytime fatigue identified in lung cancer patients can be attributed to difficulty with respiration during the night (Sandek, Andersson, Bratel, Hellstrom, Lagerstrand, 1999). While respiratory complaints are common in lung cancer patients, there are other types of cancer diagnoses that interfere with breathing (Greenberg, Gray, Mannix, Eisenthal, & Carey, 1993; Kimura, Adlakha, Staats, & Shepard, 1999; Simpson, Lee, & Cameron 1996).

Patients with obstructions to airway passage or mucosal hemangiomas may develop obstructive sleep apnea. Sleep disturbance can also be attributed to coughing and alterations in immunologic function, which in turn can be associated with changes in sleep patterns. Pain can manifest in many ways and, obviously, can disrupt sleep.

Pharmacotherapy

There are many medications that contribute to sleep problems. Graci (2005) identified common agents that may cause insomnia. The following common cancer treatment medications that can elicit or aggravate insomnia are identified but are not limited to central nervous system stimulants (e.g., amphetamines, caffeine, diet pills), sedatives and hypnotics, cancer chemotherapeutic agents, radiotherapy, anticonvulsants, adrenocorticotropins, psychotropic medications, alcohol, sedating medications (benzodiazepines, tranquilizers, illicit drugs), hormones, and decongestant medications (Kupfer & Reynolds, 1997; National Cancer Institute, 2019).

Sedating and analgesic medications (especially opioids and their derivatives) can initially assist in restoration of sleep (Lazarus, Fitzmartin, & Goldenheim, 1990) but may also contribute to sleep disruption and daytime sleepiness (Moore & Dimsdale, 2002). Benzodiazepines, although still the first-line treatment for many causes of insomnia, have potential addictive properties, including tolerance (Michelini, Cassano, Frare, & Perugi, 1996; Puntillo, Casella, & Reid, 1997). In addition, there is evidence that benzodiazepines only slightly reduce sleep latency (time to fall asleep) and significantly increase sleep duration. The concern with prescribing benzodiazepines is that discontinuation is associated with a rebound effect, where insomnia returns to higher than baseline levels for one or two nights following acute medication discontinuation. It is characterized by an increase in sleep latency onset and poor sleep efficiency (Roehrs & Roth, 2001). The immediate side effects of benzodiazepines include a next-day "hangover" effect, motor slowing, and cognitive difficulties (Holbrook, Crowther, Lotter, & Endeshaw, 2001).

Antidepressant medications may also increase the risk of twitching or jerking movements (myoclonus) or periodic leg movements that lead to sleep disruption or awakenings (Donnelly, Davis, Walsh, & Naughton, 2002). Selective serotonin reuptake inhibitors (SSRIs) and monoamine oxidase inhibitors (MAOIs) are also associated with sleep disruptions because most of these medications are classified as stimulants. Patients taking SSRIs and MAOIs have shown increases in light sleep (stage 1 and 2 sleep) and decreases in deep sleep (stage 3 and 4 sleep), as well as an increase in the time taken to enter REM sleep (Stepanski, 2002b; Walter & Golish, 2002).

Ironically, the majority of cancer patients taking these medications report improved subjective sleep quality (Oberndorfer, Saletu-Zyhlarz, & Saletu, 2000). The reasons for this discrepancy are not entirely clear. Other antidepressant medications have similar paradoxical findings (Stepanski, 2002a). Additionally, short-acting amphetamines (stimulants) are also prescribed as antidepressant agents (Stepanski, 2002a; Walter & Golish, 2002).

The effect that stimulant medications can improve sleep is unexpected because the prescription of stimulants would be contraindicated in insomnia, as this class of medications is known to disrupt sleep cycles. However, used judiciously, stimulants may have a positive effect on sleep by treating daytime fatigue and sedation. If patients can maintain alertness during the day, they are less likely to nap and, therefore, more likely to sleep at night. To achieve this effect, the stimulant should be given in small doses, early in the day.

Chemotherapy and Radiation Treatment

Cancer chemotherapy, in general, and antimetabolites and cytotoxic agents, in particular, are associated with sleep disruption (Broeckel, Jacobsen, Horton, Balducci, & Lyman, 1998; Owen, Parker, & McGuire, 1999) and greater fatigue during the daytime (Berger, 1997; Berger & Farr, 1999) Radiation therapy is also commonly associated with increased sleep disturbance, increases in daytime fatigue, and somnolence, as well as higher levels of daytime dysfunction (Irwin, Smith, & Gillin, 1992). If patients are kept awake during the night from nausea and vomiting and/or pain, they will be sleepy during the day. Napping to restore sleep loss from the previous night will only compound the difficulty of trying to fall asleep and maintain sleep throughout the nocturnal period.

Sleep Assessment

Clinical interviews are extremely useful in obtaining information on the nature, history, and severity of sleep disturbance (Bastien, Vallières, & Morin, 2001; Stepanski, Rybarczyk, Lopez, & Steven, 2003). However, a trained sleep professional would need to conduct a detailed sleep evaluation. If a patient does not seek treatment from a sleep professional, a medical professional can ask sleep questions to gain further insight into the cause and timing of the sleep difficulty.

In the absence of a detailed sleep assessment, patients should be asked about the onset, timing, quantity, and quality of their sleep, as well as their level of fatigue. Examples include but are not limited to: How were you sleeping prior to your cancer diagnosis? How have you been sleeping lately? Do you have difficulty falling asleep, staying asleep, or both? and How tired have you been during the day? Additionally, the assessment should include past episodes of sleep problems, as well as possible contributing factors (e.g., stress, depression, illness, medication, pain, nausea). It should also include a list of current medications, particularly those prescribed or taken over-the-counter for sleep problems. It is important to determine whether medication-induced sleep disturbance is due to steroids, chemotherapeutic agents, inhalers, or other medications.

Patients identified with a sleep problem should be asked to monitor their sleep in the form of a sleep log. Sleep logs provide clinicians/physicians with basic information regarding patients' sleep. Depending on how detailed the sleep log is, the clinician/physician can gain tremendous insight into daily and evening behaviors and activities, stressful events, and diet and exercise information. However, sleep logs are subject to error because they are subjective ratings of sleep. It is sometimes beneficial to obtain corroborative information about sleep functioning from patients' bed partners. Last, assessing the use of alcohol, caffeine, nicotine, and daytime napping is essential in determining whether the patients' behavior is the primary determinant of sleep disturbance. Once patients are aware of behaviors that can negatively impact sleep, they are more likely to avoid these behaviors to improve their sleep functioning.

Therapeutic Approaches

Medication

Hypnotics, both benzodiazepines and non-benzodiazepines, are the class of medications most often prescribed for cancer patients. The prescribing physician needs to be cognizant about the interactions between sleep medications, age of patient, and cancer medications. These considerations affect timing of medication, duration of how long the medication is metabolized, and side effects that could further impair cancer patients, especially if they are frail from their disease burden. These types of medications can have positive and negative effects on sleep, as discussed in this chapter. Pharmacotherapy for chronic insomnia is not recommended, except on a short-term basis and as an adjunctive treatment. The possibility of a primary sleep disorder should always be ruled out prior to pharmacologic treatment. Many medical professionals are not trained in the field of sleep medicine and are more likely to prescribe sedating medication to help a patient restore sleep. The main issue is that sedating medications are taking a "Band-Aid approach" to helping the patient sleep, but they do not address the primary cause for the sleep disturbance.

Behavioral Treatment

The three general approaches to behavioral treatment (sleep hygiene, stimulus control, and sleep restriction) (Bastien, Vallieres, & Morin, 2004; Manber & Kuo, 2002), as well as common relaxation strategies are used in managing insomnia. A trained sleep provider can teach the patient any of these three behavioral treatment approaches and should be monitored for challenges and successes. Mills and Graci (2004) provide a more thorough review of behavioral and cognitive behavioral treatment strategies. After a brief educational session, the patient initiates the behaviors at home. During subsequent clinic visits, a follow-up inquiry of the success of these behaviors is warranted, as is a discussion of specific barriers to achieving the goals of treatment. All three require that patients monitor their sleep patterns as they initiate these changes while monitoring their sleep, rest, and wake times using a sleep self-monitoring form or other assessment instrument.

If patients are exhibiting anxiety, they are likely to benefit from relaxation techniques. These range from relatively simple techniques that require three to five minutes of teaching to much more complex shifts in patients' view of life, which may require two months or more of teaching. Some of these techniques are progressive muscle relaxation, biofeedback, and guided imagery and will require a trained professional to teach. Additionally, anxiety and depression are common reactions to receiving a diagnosis of cancer. The clinician needs to address the anxiety and/or depression so that the behavioral techniques that are utilized will assist in not only improving sleep but also promote relaxation.

Cognitive Behavioral Therapy

In addition to these three specific strategies, a more general cognitive behavioral approach is implemented. For example, many patients who have difficulty sleeping begin to worry about their lack of sleep and the nightly struggle to achieve restful sleep. They may ruminate more about their sleep patterns than the current psychosocial stressors they are experiencing. They begin to develop cognitions that only amplify the problem. Sleep difficulties may be potential contributors to ongoing problems.

Although cognitive behavioral treatment has established efficacy in treating both short-term and long-term insomnia, it is "time-invasive," because many cancer patients want their sleep restored as soon as possible and do not want to wait several weeks for sleep improvement. The patient has to put in effort with this type of therapy and address psychological and emotional issues that may be unconscious or conscious contributors to sleep disturbance. Cognitive behavioral treatment is highly recommended for long-term insomnia associated with psychologic and/or behavioral components.

Stepanski, Zorick, and Roth (1991) suggest that once it is determined that a hypnotic medication should be part of the treatment plan, medical providers should follow a series of steps to most effectively choose a therapy. For instance, what are the absorption, half-life, dosage, and chronicity of the medication? Providers should dictate a specific plan regarding frequency and timing of medication, patients should never dose escalate a drug without physician approval, and patients should be monitored for compliance and sleep habits. Additionally, consider tapering and/or withdrawing medication once a sustained therapeutic point has been achieved. A general rule of thumb is to prescribe medications for short-term use (i.e., no more than three to four weeks) and be aware of rebound insomnia following discontinuation (Kupfer & Reynolds, 1997).

Some cancer patients may be either too weak or fatigued to attend face-to-face appointments or may not be able to drive due to their illness. We do not want the physical limitations of patients to impact their ability to psychosocial, behavioral, cognitive behavioral, or sleep therapy appointments. It is suggested that clinical appointments are scheduled for the same day a patient is going to an oncology clinic and/or scheduling days of therapy when the patient may feel the strongest. When patients are receiving cancer treatment, there may be days of the week or month when they feel the worst. The clinician is strongly advised to not schedule appointments during these times. Last, there is always the option of utilizing telemedicine video or telephone appointments in certain cases.

Conclusion

The cause of chronic sleep difficulties is multifaceted, and until recently, little attention has been given to the pathogenesis of cancer-related insomnia. Educating patients and health professionals about sleep is important yet often overlooked. Clinicians need to inquire about the nature, duration, and severity of the insomnia complaint and determine how these factors contribute to the onset and maintenance of insomnia.

Cancer patients are often reluctant to raise the question of sleep with their physicians or other health care providers (Graci, 2005; Engstrom,

Strohl, Rose, Lewandowski, & Stefanek, 1999; Mills & Graci, 2004). Therefore, unless the nurse or physician directly inquires about sleep disturbance, the issue is likely to remain unaddressed. Nurses, physicians, and other health care providers are in a unique position to greatly improve the quality of sleep in cancer patients. The overarching objective of treating insomnia complaints is to improve daily functioning and increase quality-of-life ratings. Cancer patients face many challenges; sleep problems do not have to be one of them.

The following case scenarios provide an illustrative review of cancer diagnoses and how the disease and/or treatment can interact with psychological functioning to affect sleep. There is no simple treatment that restores sleep. Often the clinician has to consider all the factors that are affecting the patient and tease them out to determine if the disease, psychological adaptation to being given a life-threatening diagnosis, and/or side effects of medications impact sleep. A thorough intake will review sleep history, medical history, medication (prescription and nonprescription) including vitamins and herbal supplements, psychological functioning, stressors, pain, and so on. The intake can be time-consuming, but all activities and factors of a patient's life may provide important information regarding diagnosis and treatment.

Case Study: Rumination about Dying in Sleep

Janet was a sixty-two-year-old single, retired, female who was diagnosed with acute myeloid leukemia (AML) and had been hospitalized for the last two months. She was informed that her bone marrow treatment failed. Her AML was rapidly progressing, as was her decline in overall health. Janet was referred by the bone marrow unit because she refused to sleep and had not slept in the past three nights. She was described as highly anxious and tried to walk the hallway at night because she wanted to stay awake, but she was unable to independently walk.

Janet was interviewed and she stated that she is "afraid to fall asleep because her heart might stop beating." She had no history of heart disease, and review of her medical chart did not indicate that she was experiencing heart failure.

The intake session lasted for two hours, and Janet strongly empathized that she wanted to live for her daughter and grandchildren. She was afraid that if she fell asleep, she would pass away in her sleep and miss out on living. When asked what it would take to prove to her that her heart was not weak, she stated that she was not sure.

Due to the urgency of this situation and the need for the patient to relax and rest, the treating clinician triaged with cardiology and reviewed

Janet's case. A plan was implemented in which the cardiologist would have an electrocardiogram (ECG) done and have a discussion regarding the findings as they pertained to Janet's health.

An ECG machine was brought into Janet's room, and the results were reviewed with her. The ECG summary showed that Janet had normal sinus rhythm. The cardiologist listened to her heart and told her that her heart was functioning normally. He also showed her the ECG printout, which stated normal sinus rhythm. She looked at the cardiologist, wide-eyed, and said, "My heart is okay? I can go to sleep and not fear that I won't wake up?" The cardiologist reiterated that her heart was functioning normally and that she needed her energy and strength to help her body to help fight her cancer.

This case scenario illustrates that sometimes the clinician has to try to find a solution that is not dependent on multiple follow-up appointments, sleep restriction treatment, completing sleep logs, implementing adaptive sleep hygiene behaviors, and so on. If the clinician was to engage in cognitive behavioral therapy (CBT) and try to challenge Janet's faulty belief regarding the health status of her heart, it could have taken days/weeks to see a sleep improvement. Showing her the evidence that her heart was functioning within normal limits was beneficial because Janet could not refute the evidence. Sometimes, the clinician has to think outside the box in terms of finding the best treatment regimen for the patient.

Janet was referred to a psychologist to deal with end-of-life issues and other factors associated with her declining health status. Three weeks after the cardiology intervention, Janet passed away. However, during those three weeks, she spent quality time with her daughter and grandchildren.

Case Study: Treatment of a Substance-Induced Sleep Disorder

Liz, a thirty-one-year-old married architect was referred by her medical oncologist for disordered sleep. On interview, she looked emotionally distressed and tired. She stated that she never had difficulty falling or staying asleep until her diagnosis of stage 3 metastatic breast cancer. Her treatment was undergoing chemotherapy and radiation, followed by a bilateral mastectomy. After the surgery, her husband told her that he was filing for divorce. They had two children, aged four and seven years old. She had difficulty focusing during the day because she was having difficulties falling asleep and staying asleep. She lay in bed worrying about her health, her children, and the fact that her husband did not "want to be married to a woman without breasts." She denied a psychiatric history but endorsed experiencing anxiety because she was having difficulty sleeping.

Liz's sleep difficulties began when she was prescribed a medication that caused hot flashes. She stated that because she could not sleep due to the hot flashes, she ruminated about her current health status and the welfare of her children "because there is nothing else to do at night." Her current hot flash medication was discontinued, and her sleep disturbance dissipated within one to two weeks.

While she reported being "brokenhearted" that her husband could not remain married to a woman without breasts, she did not want to be in a relationship with someone that superficial. She attended a support group for breast cancer survivors and found it to be very beneficial. She started another hot flash medication that did not have insomnia/sleep disturbance side effects and has reported no sleep disturbance issues.

Case Study: Treatment of Pain

Walter, a sixty-seven-year-old, married, retired architect, was referred by his oncologist for difficulty maintaining sleep. He had significant back pain, weight loss, and fatigue. He went to his general practitioner, who referred him to an oncologist. Walter stated that he was initially diagnosed with stage 3 multiple myeloma. He recently fractured his rib but was unsure how it happened. The "bone pain" was constant, and his medical oncologist prescribed opioid medication (fentanyl) that "tapered the pain," but it remained.

He stated that he takes his pain medication one hour before going to bed (9:00 p.m.) and usually had no difficulty falling asleep. He reported that he woke up at approximately 1:00 a.m. with back pain and was unable to fall back asleep. He reported the "breakthrough pain" to his oncologist, and they made medication and dosage changes with no success.

Walter appeared to engage in good sleep hygiene behaviors with scheduled bedtime and wake times. He denied a significant psychological history.

A review of his medications revealed that none of the medications caused sleep disturbance. He was referred to the pain clinic to address his pain. He was given a sleep log to complete and was asked to return in two weeks.

Walter returned with two weeks of sleep-log data. He scheduled an appointment within three days to the pain service clinic, and the physician changed his pain medications and included a slow-acting opioid to address the breakthrough pain. The first three days of sleep-log data showed poor sleep efficiency (72%), and after he started his new medication, his sleep efficiency improved to 93%.

He was asked to continue completing the sleep logs for another three weeks and return for a follow-up visit. Review of his three-week sleep log showed that he continued to report not experiencing sleep maintenance issues. He woke up to urinate one or two times per night, but he was able to quickly return to sleep. His sleep efficiency remained above 90%. He reported being satisfied with his sleep regime. Walter also stated that he was not aware that specialty pain clinics exist; he was "happy" that his pain was being controlled and that he could enjoy life and not be reminded every minute that he had cancer. While he remained fatigued from his cancer, he reported an increase in quality of life because his sleep had been restored.

References

M. Aldrich (2000). Cardinal manifestations of sleep disorders. In M. H. Kryger, T. Roth, & W. C. Dement (Eds.), *Principles and practice of sleep medicine* (526–528). Philadelphia, PA: WB Saunders.

American Academy of Sleep Medicine (2001). *International classification of sleep disorders, revised diagnostic and coding manual.* Westchester, IL: American Academy of Sleep Medicine.

American Psychiatric Association (2013). *Diagnostic and statistical manual of mental disorders* (5th ed.). Arlington, VA: American Psychiatric Publishing.

C. H. Bastien, A. Vallieres, & C. M. Morin (2001). Validation of the Insomnia Severity Index as an outcome measure for insomnia research. *Sleep Medicine, 2*, 297–307.

C. H. Bastien, A. Vallieres, & C. M. Morin (2004). Precipitating factors of insomnia. *Behavioral Sleep Medicine, 2*, 50–62.

R. M. Benca (2001). Consequences of insomnia and its therapies. *Journal of Clinical Psychiatry, 62* (Suppl. 10), 33–38.

A. M. Berger (1997). *Patterns of fatigue and factors influencing fatigue during adjuvant breast cancer chemotherapy* (dissertation). Omaha: University of Nebraska Medical Center.

A. M. Berger, & L. Farr (1999). The influence of daytime inactivity and nighttime restlessness on cancer-related fatigue. *Oncology Nursing Forum, 26*, 1663–1671.

J. A. Broeckel, P. B. Jacobsen, J. Horton, L. Balducci, & G. H. Lyman (1998). Characteristics and correlates of fatigue after adjuvant chemotherapy for breast cancer. *Journal of Clinical Oncology, 16*:1689–1696.

R. J. Couzi, K. J. Helzlsouer, & J. H. Fetting (1995). Prevalence of menopausal symptoms among women with a history of breast cancer and attitudes toward estrogen replacement therapy. *Journal of Clinical Oncology, 13*, 2737–2744.

J. R. Davidson, A. W. MacLean, M. D. Brundage, & K. Schulze (2002). Sleep disturbance in cancer patients. *Social Science Medicine, 54*:1309–1321.

S. Donnelly, M. P. Davis, D, Walsh, & M. Naughton (2002). Morphine in cancer pain management: A practical guide. *Support Care Cancer, 10*, 13–35.

B. Ehrenberg (2000). Importance of sleep restoration in co-morbid disease: Effect of anticonvulsants. *Neurology, 54*(5 Suppl. 1), S33–S37.

C. A. Engstrom, R. A. Strohl, L. Rose, L. Lewandowski, & M. E. Stefanek (1999). Sleep alterations in cancer patients. *Cancer Nursing, 22*, 143–148.

B. V. Fortner, E. J. Stepanski, S. C. Wang, S. Kasprowicz, & H. H. Durrence (2002). Sleep and quality of life in breast cancer patients. *Journal of Pain and Symptom Management, 24*, 471–480.

G. M. Graci (2005). Pathogenesis and management of cancer-related insomnia. *Journal of Supportive Oncology, 3*(5), 349–359.

D. B. Greenberg, J. L. Gray, C. M. Mannix, S. Eisenthal, & M. Carey (1993). Treatment-related fatigue and serum interleukin-1 levels in patients during external beam irradiation for prostate cancer. *Journal of Pain and Symptom Management, 8*, 196–200.

A. Holbrook, R. Crowther, A. Lotter, & Y. Endeshaw (2001). The role of benzodiazepines in the treatment of insomnia: Meta-analysis of benzodiazepine use in the treatment of insomnia. *Journal of the American Geriatrics Society, 49*, 824–826.

A. M. Holbrook, R. Crowther, A. Lotter, C. Cheng, & D. King (2000a). The diagnosis and management of insomnia in clinical practice: A practical evidence-based approach. *CMAJ, 162*, 216–220.

A. M. Holbrook, R. Crowther, A. Lotter, C. Cheng, & D. King (2000b). Meta-analysis of benzodiazepine use in the treatment of insomnia. *CMAJ, 162*, 225–233.

M. Irwin, T. L. Smith, & J. C. Gillin (1992). Electroencepha-lographic sleep and natural killer activity in depressed patients and control subjects. *Psychosomatic Medicine, 54*, 10–21.

S. Jacobs-Rebhun, P. P. Schnurr, M. J. Friedman, R. Peck, M. Brophy, & D. Fuller (2000). Posttraumatic stress disorder and sleep difficulty. *American Journal of Psychiatry, 157*, 1525–1526.

K. Kimura, A. Adlakha, B. A. Staats, & J. W. Shepard, Jr. (1999). Successful treatment of obstructive sleep apnea with use of nasal continuous positive airway pressure in three patients with mucosal hemangiomas of the oral cavity. *Mayo Clinic Proceedings, 74*, 155–158.

D. J. Kupfer, & C. F. Reynolds (1997). Management of insomnia. *New England Journal of Medicine, 336*, 341–346.

H. Lazarus, R. D. Fitzmartin, & P. D. Goldenheim (1990). A multi-investigator clinical evaluation of oral controlled-release morphine (MS Contin tablets) administered to cancer patients. *Hospice Journal, 6*, 1–15.

D. Leger, C. Guilleminault, J. P. Dreyfus, C. Delahaye, & M. Paillard (2000). Prevalence of insomnia in a survey of 12,778 adults in France. *Journal of Sleep Research, 9*, 35–42.

C. Lindley, S. Vasa, W. T. Sawyer, & E. P. Winer (1998). Quality of life and preferences for treatment following systemic adjuvant therapy for early-stage breast cancer. *Journal of Clinical Oncology, 16*, 1380–1387.

R. Manber, & T. Kuo (2002). Cognitive-behavioral therapies for insomnia. In T. L. Lee-Chiong, Jr., M. Sateia, & M. Carskadon (Eds.), *Sleep medicine* (pp. 177–185). Philadelphia, PA: Hanley & Belfus Inc.

M. J. Massie, & M. K. Popkin. (1998). Depressive disorders. In J.C. Holland (Ed.), *Psycho-oncology* (pp. 518). New York: Oxford University Press.

S. Michelini, G. B. Cassano, F. Frare, & G. Perugi (1996). Long-term use of benzodiazepines: Tolerance, dependence and clinical problems in anxiety and mood disorders. *Pharmacopsychiatry, 29*, 127–134.

M. Mills, & G. Graci (2004). Sleep disturbances. In M. Frogge (Ed.), *Cancer symptom management* (111–134). Sudbury, MA: Jones & Bartlett Publishers.

P. Moore, & J. E. Dimsdale (2002). Opioids, sleep, and cancer-related fatigue. *Medical Hypotheses, 58*, 77–82.

C. M. Morin (2000). The nature of insomnia and the need to refine our diagnostic criteria. *Psychosomatic Medicine, 62*, 483–485.

National Cancer Institute. *Sleep disorders*. Retrieved July 22, 2019, from: http://www.nci.nih.gov/cancertopics/pdq/supportivecare/sleepdisorders/patient/allpages

R. Noyes, C. Holt, & M. Massie (1998). Anxiety disorders. In J. Holland (Ed.), *Psycho-oncology* (pp. 548–563). New York: Oxford University Press.

S. Oberndorfer, G. Saletu-Zyhlarz, & B. Saletu (2000). Effects of selective serotonin reuptake inhibitors on objective and subjective sleep quality. *Neuropsychobiology, 42*, 69–81.

M. M. Ohayon, M. Caulet, R. G. Priest, & C. Guilleminault (1997). DSM-IV and ICSD-90 insomnia symptoms and sleep dissatisfaction. *British Journal of Psychiatry, 171*, 382–388.

M. Omne-Pontén, L. Holmberg, T. Burns, H. O. Adami, & R. Bergstrom (1992). Determinants of the psycho-social outcome after operation for breast cancer. Results of a prospective comparative interview study following mastectomy and breast conservation. *European Journal of Cancer, 28A*(6–7), 1062–1067. https://doi.org/10.1016/0959-8049(92)90457-d

D. C. Owen, K. P. Parker, & D. B. McGuire (1999). Comparison of subjective sleep quality in patients with cancer and healthy subjects. *Oncology Nursing Forum, 26*, 1649–1651.

S. D. Passik, L. A. Whitcomb, K. L. Kirsh, & D. E. Theobald (2003). An unsuccessful attempt to develop a single-item screen for insomnia in cancer patients. *Journal of Pain and Symptom Management, 25*, 284–287.

K. Puntillo, V. Casella, & M. Reid (1997). Opioid and benzodiazepine tolerance and dependence: Application of theory to critical care practice. *Heart & Lung, 26*, 317–324.

T. Roehrs, & T. Roth (2016). Hypnotics: Efficacy and adverse effects. In M. H. Kryger, T. Roth, W. C. Dement (Eds.), *Principles and practice of sleep medicine* (pp. 414–418). Philadelphia, PA: WB Saunders.

T. Roth, & S. Ancoli-Israel (1999). Daytime consequences and correlates of insomnia in the United States: Results of the 1991 National Sleep Foundation Survey. II. *Sleep, 22*(Suppl. 2), S354–S358.

K. Sandek, T. Andersson, T. Bratel, G. Hellstrom, & L. Lagerstrand (1999). Sleep quality, carbon dioxide responsiveness and hypoxaemic patterns in nocturnal hypoxaemia due to chronic obstructive pulmonary disease (COPD) without daytime hypoxaemia. *Respiratory Medicine, 93*, 79–87.

J. Savard, H. Ivers, M. Savard, & C. M. Morin (2016). Long-term effects of two formats of CBT for insomnia comorbid with breast cancer. *Sleep, 39*(4), 813–823.

J. Savard, S. M. Miller, M. Mills, A. O'Leary, H. Harding, S. Douglas, C. Mangan, R. Belch, & A. Winokur (1999). Association between subjective sleep quality and depression on immunocompetence in low-income women at risk for cervical cancer. *Psychosomatic Medicine, 61*, 496–507.

J. Savard, & C. M. Morin (2001). Insomnia in the context of cancer: A review of a neglected problem. *Journal of Clinical Oncology, 19*, 895–908.

J. Savard, S. Simard, J. Blanchet, H. Ivers, & C. M. Morin (2001). Prevalence, clinical characteristics, and risk factors for insomnia in the context of breast cancer. *Sleep, 24*, 583–590.

P. M. Silberfarb, P. J. Hauri, T. E. Oxman, & P. Schnurr (1993). Assessment of sleep in patients with lung cancer and breast cancer. *Journal of Clinical Oncology, 11*, 997–1004.

T. Simpson, E. R. Lee, & C. Cameron. Patients' perceptions of environmental factors that disturb sleep after cardiac surgery. *American Journal of Critical Care, 5*, 173–181.

E. Stepanski (2002a). Etiology of insomnia. In T. L. Lee-Chiong, Jr., M. Sateia, & M. Carskadon (Eds.), *Sleep medicine* (pp. 161–168). Philadelphia, PA: Hanley & Belfus Inc.

E. Stepanski, B. Rybarczyk, M. Lopez, & S. Steven (2003). Assessment and treatment of sleep disorders in older adults: A review for rehabilitation psychologists. *Rehabilitation Psychology, 48*, 23–36.

E. Stepanski, F. Zorick, & T. Roth (1991). Pharmacotherapy of insomnia. In P. J. Hauri (Ed.), *Case Studies in Insomnia*. Critical Issues in Psychiatry (pp. 115–129). New York: Plenum Publishing.

E. J. Stepanski (2002b). The effect of sleep fragmentation on daytime function. *Sleep, 25*, 268–276.

A. van't Spijker, R. W. Trijsburg, & H. J. Duivenvoorden (1997). Psychological sequelae of cancer diagnosis: A meta-analytical review of 58 studies after 1980. *Psychosomatic Medicine, 59*, 280–293.

T. Walter, & J. Golish (2002). Psychotropic and neurologic medications. In T. L. Lee-Chiong, Jr., M. Sateia, & M. Carskadon (Eds.), *Sleep medicine* (pp. 587–599). Philadelphia, PA: Hanley & Belfus Inc.

Y. Wengstrom, C. Haggmark, H. Strander, & C. Forsberg (2000). Perceived symptoms and quality of life in women with breast cancer receiving radiation therapy. *European Journal of Oncology Nursing, 4*, 78–88.

CHAPTER 10

Dreaming as a Psychological Process

Why do we dream, why are some dreams frightening, and why do we only remember some of our dreams? Hypotheses have abounded for years regarding the meaning and biological or neurological pathway of dreams. Some people earn a living by analyzing dreams, but what do dreams really mean, and what is the current dream landscape? The symbolic meaning of dreams is called the latent content of dreams, and many people believe there are hidden messages in dreams. Some scientists believe that dreaming is related to depression, and some therapists postulate that if the unconscious meaning of dreams can be interpreted, then psychological distress could be relieved (Cherry, 2020). This chapter will explore dreaming as a psychological process.

A dream is defined as a physiologically and psychologically conscious state that occurs during sleep. It is often characterized by a rich array of endogenous sensory, motor, emotional, and other experiences (American Psychological Association [APA], 2020). Dreams mainly occur in rapid eye movement (REM) sleep and may be logical or illogical. Dream interpretation is the attempt at finding meaning from dreams as it applies to an individual's life.

Sigmund Freud believed that the meaning and content of dreams were heavily encrypted and hard to translate (Lyon, 1990). The hidden meaning of dreams played an important role in Freud's psychoanalytic theory, and he believed that bringing the hidden meaning of a dream into conscious awareness could relieve psychological distress (Freud, 1913). For instance, Freud believed that the latent content of a dream was not only suppressed but hidden by the subconscious mind to protect the person from thoughts and feelings that were hard to cope with (Cherry, 2020).

While the function of sleep is hypothezied to be based on restorative properties, there is no concluding evidence that this is true. The early work of Dr. Rosalind Cartwright (the Grandmother of Sleep) showed the scientific measurement of sleep and dreaming, primarily dreams and the process of dreaming. "Dreams," wrote Cartwright, "are our private perceptions which cannot be validated or shared by others" (Cartwright, 1977). She also postulated that dreams may "provide us with a direct cure for certain mental problems long before anyone determines exactly what sleep and dreaming are for" (Lyon, 1990).

The history of dreams has been reported by the early Greeks, ancient Egyptians, and Romans, who believed that dreams came from an external source—gods speaking to humans, either influencing the person or others (Learning English: Explorations, 2016). To the ancient Egyptians, dreams were times of forecasting and being spoken to in prophecies. In Cleopatra's time, there were "dream schools." Remains of dream diaries on papyrus have been excavated detailing recordings of dreams. These historical accountings underscore the visionary narrative of the dream and dreaming to the dreamer.

Some of the first laboratory experiments developed by Dr. Cartwright involved brain wave measurement during sleep, which included periods of rapid eye movement dream sleep (Cartwright, 1977). In addition, a presentation of photos or a communication from the experimenter was presented to the participant before sleep, with a measurement of recall. These fundamental studies formed the foundation of understanding the information processing role of dream sleep.

HuffPost (2017), in an online sleep article, stated that Rubin Naiman, a sleep and dream expert on the clinical faculty of the Arizona Center for Integrative Medicine, believes, "Good dreaming contributes to our psychological well-being by supporting healthy memory, warding off depression, and expanding our ordinary limited consciousness into broader, spiritual realms." Furthermore, a study at Harvard Medical School (2012) revealed that dreaming also helps consolidate memories and retain information.

Dr. Cartwright (2010), in her sleep and dream research, states the following:

> The more severe the depression, the earlier the first REM begins. Sometimes it starts as early as 45 minutes into sleep. That means these sleepers' first cycle of NREM sleep amounts to about half the

usual length of time. This early REM displaces the initial deep sleep, which is not fully recovered later in the night. This displacement of the first deep sleep is accompanied by an absence of the usual large outflow of growth hormone. The timing of the greatest release of human growth hormone (HGH) is in the first deep sleep cycle. The depressed have very little SWS [slow-wave sleep, stages 3 and 4 of the sleep cycle] and no big pulse of HGH; and in addition to growth, HGH is related to physical repair. If we do not get enough deep sleep, our bodies take longer to heal and grow. The absence of the large spurt of HGH during the first deep sleep continues in many depressed patients even when they are no longer depressed (in remission). The first REM sleep period not only begins too early in the night in people who are clinically depressed, it is also often abnormally long. Instead of the usual 10 minutes or so, this REM may last twice that. The eye movements too are abnormal—either too sparse or too dense. In fact, they are sometimes so frequent that they are called *eye movement storms*.

Interestingly, what has perplexed sleep-dream researchers is that when depressed subjects are awakened five minutes into their first REM sleep episode, they have no recall of what they were "experiencing" (Popova, 2019). This finding has been repeated by sleep-dream researchers, and there is no clear understanding of what is occurring. If antidepressants suppress REM sleep (reducing the time in REM sleep), is this responsible for mood elevation in the depressed? It is not really clear to researchers.

As a person sleeps throughout the night, the sleep cycles transition from light sleep, to deep sleep, to REM—dream sleep, and then back to light sleep, deep sleep, and another dream episode (REM sleep). We have about four cycles of sleep each night. We may spend more time in light sleep (stages 1 and 2) than deep (slow wave) or REM sleep, and our sleep cycles change as we mature from infancy to older age.

Moss (2009) reported measurable changes in consciousness during wake and dreaming. Klein (2018) proposed that the dream narrative originates with the dreamer—that environmental or social influences do not provide an identity to the dream. Lloyd and Cartwright (1995) originally proposed that one's subjective experiences are projected in the personal perception of the dream. Dream collections taken from home dream logs and dream reportings once subjects were awakened in the sleep laboratory were not distinguishable.

Cartwright's original research was in-line with dream content analysis researchers such as Hall and Vander Castle in the study of dreams. Olsen,

Schnell, and Carlsson (2016) further examined the subjective experience in the dream with a statistical analysis of dream content. Dreams are considered to have meaningful information processing (memory consolidation, sorting inputs, and solving problems), a forecast/prophecy component, and neural products of the brain.

LaBerge's study of lucid dreaming (i.e., becoming conscious enough to know that dreaming is occurring) provided the scientific and clinical communities with a broader conceptuality of the features of dreaming. Lucid dreams are when the dreamers become aware of themselves dreaming and place themselves into the dream to broaden, deepen, correct, or perform many other functions of the dream. Klein (2018) identified the therapeutic gains of lucid dreaming for patients with posttraumatic stress disorder. Increases in dream content were found following therapeutic instructions to lucid dream. Last, Foulkes (1977) identified the qualitative difference in dreams of children and adults. The mental state of consciousness differs between the children and adult groups due to life experience, accounting for the variable difference.

Dreams induced during hypnotherapy sessions can be therapeutic. Graci (2010) noted that hypnotists may suggest that the patient have a dream during hypnotherapy sessions, with a similar content to a daydream or night dream. The therapist will use these dreams to learn about meaningful themes, problems, or conflicts (Ng & Lee, 2008). Hypnotic suggestions for nightmares or sleep terrors can include having happy, tranquil, or pleasant dreams without waking up and feeling very relaxed and calm when sleeping (De Rios & Friedman, 1990). Additional suggestions can include that when the bad dream begins, the patient try to switch to a different (more positive) dream or alter the dream content/ending (Ng & Lee, 2008; Sharma, 2007).

Graci (2010) reviews when Dr. Cartwright, the former director of the Rush Behavioral Sleep Disorders Center, during a didactic training session, discussed a case presentation of a child who experienced repeated nightmares of a frightening monster. During the session, the child was asked if he would be comfortable shaking hands with the monster and introducing himself. The child stated that he would be comfortable with talking to the monster because "when people introduce themselves, bad things don't happen." The suggestion was then given to the child that when the nightmare occurs again to approach the monster and introduce himself, ask for the monster's name, and shake hands. When the child returned for his next session, he discussed having the dream, and the monster was no longer frightening or problematic. Once the child shook hands with the monster, it was no longer frightening. The child denied having nightmares again.

Furthermore, Dr. Cartwright also suggests using alternative endings. For instance, if a patient has a recurring dream that he or she is falling or is driving an automobile and the brakes do not work, change the ending. In the case of falling, change the sequence of the dream as it occurs. For instance, an individual can suddenly have the ability to fly, which would alter the ending—he or she can be rescued (e.g., by a large object), or, when close to the ground, he or she can freeze in midair or dramatically slow the speed of decent and safely land on his or her feet. In the case of the driving with faulty brakes, change the dream so that the individual does not get into the same car or suddenly has the ability to slow the car down by inventing a magic button that can be pressed to stop the car safely (similar to a James Bond car). In either scenario, the key element is that the suggestion(s) created for individuals will foster feelings of empowerment and enhanced feelings of self-control so that he or she can create an alternative ending.

While dream research has been ongoing for a long time, there is more that needs to be learned about how dreams impact our lives and their relationship with psychological disorders. While some dreams may be frightening, others can be fun, humorous, or reflect things that occurred during our daily experiences. Dreams and memory also interact, but our memories may not actually reflect reality; memories are subjective perceptions of reality, and the content of the dreams may hold important information about our true feelings or thoughts about things.

Case Study: Dreaming and Resolving Complex Issues
Martina was a 19-year-old biology-chemistry major at a local university and experienced extreme anxiety since starting her calculus course. She stated that she did not feel as confident as her friends in taking the course; she has to spend extra time reviewing the chapter material and sometimes spent too much time trying to solve the calculus questions at the end of each chapter. She stated that her anxiety was getting the "best of her," and she was having difficulty trying to relax before bedtime.

Martina had no significant health issues, her body habitus was normal, and she denied experiencing depressive symptoms or other symptoms associated with a sleep disorder. She was asked to keep a sleep diary to determine the overall quality and quantity of sleep. She stated that she felt tired upon awakening, but once she showered and dressed, she was alert. She normally went to bed at the same time every evening, at 10:30, unless she had to stay awake to study for an exam, and she awakened at 7:30 a.m. every day. She was on the gymnastic team, so she had to be at practice by 8:00 a.m. every morning. Last, she stated that she awakened one or two times per week, generally related to a dream. When asked about the dream content/themes, she stated that the content was never the same, except if she was unable to solve a problem, such as in her calculus homework, her "mind will play out the event."

She stated that during sleep, she saw the homework question, was able to solve the problem, and awoke toward the latter part of the night. Martina wrote the solution down so that when she awoke, she had the problem solved. She stated that this "ability to solve homework problems" started when she was a freshman in high school. She generally kept a notebook on her bedside table so that she could reach for it without having to turn the light on. Last, she stated that her ability to solve problems during sleep happened for almost all her course assignments. For instance, she was enrolled in organic chemistry last semester and was able to solve the more difficult questions during dream sleep as compared to when awake. When asked what she thought caused her ability to figure out solutions during dream sleep, she stated that it was most likely due to her being much more relaxed, and her mind was "clear." She also stated that she generally woke between 3:00 and 4:00 a.m. with solutions to her homework problems.

She returned to the sleep clinic for a follow-up visit and for a review of her sleep log/journal. She noted feeling anxious in most of her science classes and was much more relaxed when attending her "nonscientific" courses. She stated that she was on scholarship and had to "get good grades," or her parents would send her home because they were unable to pay for the cost of her education plus housing.

Review of her sleep diary/journal revealed that she engaged in good sleep hygiene behaviors; she drank one iced tea per day while eating lunch and did not drink caffeinated sodas or eat chocolate. She generally ate dinner between 5:00 and 6:00 p.m. and did not exercise two to three hours before bedtime.

Her bed and wake times were consistent, and her daytime sleepiness score was within normal limits. She did not have a television in her bedroom and did not study in her bedroom. Martina described her bedroom as generally quiet and dark at night. She had a roommate, but the roommate was almost never home. Her sleep efficiency score was 92%. Most of the session focused on her inability to control her anxiety because she often felt wound up an hour before her scheduled bedtime. She also noted that she thought she was grinding her teeth during the night because she often woke with her jaw aching. The onset of the teeth grinding was when she began the calculus course. She was referred to a dentist to address the teeth grinding, as well as a psychotherapist to address her anxiety. She was given relaxation exercises to engage in prior to bedtime and was educated on adaptive sleep hygiene behaviors to assist with anxiety reduction.

A one-month up appointment revealed that she recently went to the dentist and discovered that she cracked two of her teeth from grinding her teeth during the day and while asleep. She stated that she has never had this problem before starting her calculus course. Her dentist took denture molds to create a bite plate, and she started using the new mouthpiece one week ago. She stated that it was a bit difficult to get used to, but she was doing it.

This case scenario illustrates that the mind never truly "goes to sleep" and that while some dreams may be illogical or nonsensical, dreams can serve a positive purpose. In Martina's case, her active mind was able to rest, but her unconscious mind was able to replay the homework scenarios that she had difficulty with and was able to solve the problem during dream sleep. When she awakened, she was able to record the solution to the homework assignment and reported being able to quickly return to sleep. She did not endorse daytime sleepiness and never had an injury or accident due to sleepiness. She denied all symptoms related to sleep disorders, so there was no reason to conduct an overnight sleep study. Her sleep diary/logs showed that she engaged in good sleep hygiene behaviors but was having difficulty managing her anxiety. She attended psychotherapy and learned how to control her anxiety with cognitive behavioral therapy techniques.

Case Study: Dark Dreams

Jane was a 22-year-old female PhD student who presented for psychotherapy with issues related to a dream that had been recurring since she was 8 years old. She stated that she repetitively had the same dream of a dark, large tidal wave coming at her, and there was no escaping the wave. There was no place to run or hide because her back was facing a wall, and the "wave will drown her."

Her medical history was nonsignificant, and she reported having a younger brother that she was close to. She lived with her mother and brother since her parents divorced when she was 10 years old. She stated that her parents rarely talked, and she saw her father once per month. She stated that she gets "good grades" and attended weekly group study meetings for her graduate school colleagues. She stated that she wanted to earn her PhD in counseling.

During the psychological intake, she responded positive to mildly depressed symptomology and denied experiencing anxiety, intense anger, hallucinations, disassociations, or amnesia. She stated that she often felt sad but did not know why. Generally, she appeared to be well-functioning and appropriately groomed, did not engage in high-risk behaviors, and was not suicidal.

Jane came to two intense psychotherapy sessions per week. Six months into the sessions, she discussed that she felt her father might be represented by the dark tidal wave. When queried about this thought, she stated that she did not know, but her "tidal wave dream" occurred more frequently, and the clouds were now intensely dark. She awoke when the "dark water" approached her face. The water never quite reached her, but the fear was intense, and she woke and had difficulty falling asleep. She was completing sleep logs, and review of the sleep log content showed it was identical to her recall of the dream in therapy. She stated that since therapy started, she had been avoiding her father but does not understand why.

Six months later, Jane reported that before she woke from her dream, she saw her father covering her eyes, and his hand was consistent with the wave coming toward her. She became very emotional during this session and stated that she did not know why she was crying, but she felt frightened. Therapy focused on having her process her feelings and creating a safe place for her to go to when she felt frightened.

During the next appointment, Jane revealed that she started taking yoga classes to help with the stress of graduate school so that she could unwind. She felt good after completing her yoga class—she stated that "yoga helps clear the mind and relax the body." She continued to have the same "tidal wave dream" but was unable to have any additional insight into its interpretation.

During the weekend, she called, crying hysterically stated that, "I know what happened. He did it to me." After listening to her and determining that she was not a threat to herself or anyone, she was asked to take a cab to the office for an emergency session. She was inconsolable during the session and repeatedly stated, "He molested me." Through tears and intense emotional unloading, she stated that when her yoga teacher touched her back to change the alignment of her spine to a more correct one, she had a flashback of her father touching her. Jane stated that the memories came rushing at her, and she could not control the intensity of emotion or block any of the memories.

She recalled that her father would go into her room at night and place his hand over her eyes as he began to touch her. The sexual molestation occurred when she was 8–10 years old and she moved in with her mother. She stated that her mother was an emergency-room doctor and often worked in the evening, which left her father to take care of her and her brother. She cried out, "The hand was the dark tidal wave coming at me. How could he do that to a child?"

For the next year, therapy focused on coming to terms with the sexual abuse and finding ways to move on. She took a semester off from graduate school to work on herself and to attend therapy. At the end of therapy, she stated that while her conscious mind had "hid" the trauma, her unconscious mind would not let it go. Once she was able to recall the trauma, she denied ever having another "tidal wave dream." This case scenario is an example of how the unconscious mind never stops working, and while the conscious mind may not want to recall events, the mind never really falls to sleep.

Case Study: The Fiery Phoenix

Jackson was a 38-year-old engineer who was recently terminated from his position. He presented for "treatment" for a recurring dream that started within a week of being wrongfully terminated as an engineering project lead for an international company. He stated that someone "stole" his designs and the "thief" presented them at a major president- and vice-president-level meeting. This thief was a former friend and colleague who had access to his office and computer. When Jackson tried to show that the work really was from his creativity, he was unable to find any documentation on his computer or files. His hard drive had been "wiped clean." Jackson's manager believed the colleague, and Jackson was asked to leave the company.

He reported being a happily married man (he married his college girlfriend), and they have two children, aged 12 and 8 years old. He denied a significant medical or psychiatric history.

He stated that the goal of therapy was to stop the dreams from recurring and/or to understand why the dream was occurring. He stated that in his dream, he is sitting in his office on the twelfth floor when suddenly an extremely large "fiery Phoenix bird" emerges from the parking lot. The bird turns into a "humongous" big yellow bird that is so large that he cannot even walk, and it turns to walk toward him and "get him." When asked what he thinks the dream meant, Jackson stated that he thought he was the fiery bird because the flames represent his being blacklisted in the engineering firms and that his career went up in flames. He did not know what the transformation of the Phoenix into the big yellow bird meant. Jackson was instructed that if the dream recurred, he was to change the direction of the big bird so that it walked away.

When Jackson returned for therapy one week later, he stated that he had not had the dream again and wanted to continue focusing on the dream. When asked what the "big bird" could stand for or represent in his life, he was very quiet and did not speak for 10 minutes. When he did speak, he spoke very softly and stated that, as a child, he loved the Big Bird character on *Sesame Street* and had a Big Bird doll that he took everywhere with him. Jackson was then asked, "What role does Big Bird have in your dream?" Again, silence. He appeared to be contemplating the significance of Big Bird. After some reflection, Jackson said that the Phoenix bursting in flames was his career "blowing up," and the transformation to Big Bird was significant in that it brought back childhood. Big Bird represented childhood and having to learn to grow up or start over. He was interpreting that the big bird was coming to get him but "it was probably me just trying to reach out for the safety and security I felt as a child especially when I held Big Bird." Jackson had significant clinical insight into how his waking life related to his dream content. The therapist asked thought-provoking questions, which led him to have his aha moment, where the meaning of the dream held significance to him. He never had the dream again. He attended three more sessions and reported at the last session that he found a better job working for the competitor of his former company.

Generally, psychotherapy cases and dream interpretation are not this straightforward. Jackson was a motivated, highly intelligent man with good clinical insight, and he was able to come to terms with the anxiety that he was experiencing in his dream. Once the goal of therapy had been accomplished (i.e., reducing the anxiety and stopping the recurring dream), Jackson denied having any additional psychosocial stressors in his life, and he appeared to have a healthy emotional well-being. While it is helpful for therapists, physicians, and clinicians to understand the principles of sleep, especially dreaming, this is not always the case. For those treating patients with recurring dreams, it is important to work with them on understanding the dreams without doing all the work of trying to interpret it. Clinical insight may take time, but the therapist is encouraged to "guide" the patient toward anxiety reduction, giving the proper instruction in how to address the negative occurrence in the dream (such as the child asking the monster what its first name is) so that the theme of the dream can go from frightening and anxiety-provoking to more neutral. The therapist can always instruct the patient to go back into the dream and change the ending or empower the patient to change the dream sequence or ending as he or she is dreaming. Most patients do not feel strong or empowered enough to change the outcome of the dream, but it is helpful for the therapist to provide the patient with permission to change the beginning, middle, or ending of a dream. Not all dreams have meaning, and some are simply nonsensible or illogical. In the case of Jane and her recurring dark dream of tidal waves, it did not make sense to her because she did not live by the water and did not understand how it applied to her. She only knew that it was frightening. Sometimes dream analysis, similar to psychoanalysis, can take years before progress is made. Not all dreams will have meaning, but it is important to explore them with patients, if applicable.

References

American Psychological Association (2020). *APA dictionary of psychology*. Retrieved January 3, 2020, from, https://dictionary.apa.org/dream referenced

E. J. Bayley, T. E. Fuller-Rowell, E. K. Saini, L. E. Philbrook, & M. El-Sheikh (2018). Neighborhood economic deprivation and social fragmentation associated with children's sleep. *Behavioral Sleep Medicine, 16*(6), 542–552. https://doi.org/10.1080/15402002.2016.1253011

R. D. Cartwright (1977). *Night life explorations in dreaming.* Trentin, NJ: Prentice-Hall, Inc.

R. D. Cartwright (2010). *The twenty-four hour mind: The role of sleep and dreaming in our emotional lives.* London: Oxford University Press.

K. Cherry (2020). Latent content as the hidden meaning of your dreams. *Verywell Mind.* Retrieved March 19, 2020, from, https://www.verywellmind.com/what-is-latent-content-2795330

M. Csikszentmihalyi (1996). *Creativity: Flow and the psychology of discovery and intervention.* New York: HarperCollins.

M. De Rios, & J. Friedman (1990). Suggestions when there are sleep problems. In D. Hammond (Ed.), *Handbook of hypnotic suggestions and metaphors* (p. 337). New York: W.W. Norton & Company.

G. Delaney (1991). *Breakthrough dreaming: How to tap the power of your 24-hours mind.* New York: Bantam Press.

R. Ferber (1985). *Solve your child's sleep problems.* New York: Fireside Books.

D. Foulkes (1977). Children's dreams: Age changes and sex differences. *Waking and Sleeping, 1*(2), 171–174.

S. Freud (1913). *The interpretation of dreams.* (3rd ed., A. A. Brill, trans.). New York: The Macmillan Company (Bartleby.com, 2010).

G. Graci (2010). Hypnotherapy and parasomnias. In M. J. Thorpy & G. Plazzi (Eds.), *The Parasomnias and other sleep-related movement disorders* (pp. 338–344). Cambridge, MA: Cambridge University Press.

Harvard Medical School (2012, February). Learning while you sleep: Dream or Reality? Harvard Health Publishing. Retrieved April 21, 2021, from www.health.harvard.edu/staying-healthy/learning-while-you-sleep.

M. Hauan, L. Strand, & L. E Laugsand (2018). Associations of insomnia symptoms with blood pressure and resting heart rate: The Hunt Study in Norway. *Behavioral Sleep Medicine, 16*(5), 504–522. https://doi.org/10.1080/15402002.2016.1228651

HuffPost (2017). *What do your dreams say about your sleep quality.* Retrieved September 18, 2018, from, https://www.huffpost.com/entry/dreams-sleep-quality_n_8513908

S. B. Klein (2018). The phenomenology of REM-sleep dreaming: The contributions of personal and perspectival ownership, subjective temporality, and episodic memory. *Psychology of Consciousness: Theory, Research and Practice, 6*(1), 55–66. https://doi.org/10.1037/cns0000174.

S. LaBerge (1990). Lucid dreaming: Psychophysiological studies of consciousness during REM sleep. In R. R. Bootzen, J. F. Kihlstrom, & D. L. Schacter (Eds.), *Sleep and cognition* (109–126). Washington, DC: American Psychological Association

J. D. Lamoreaux (2002). *The early Muslim tradition of dream interpretation.* Albany: State University of New York Press.

LearningEnglish:Explorations(2016). *Sleep science:The mystery of dreams and dreaming.* https://learningenglish.voanews.com/a/a-23-2009-05-19-voa1-83141262/129734.html

J. Lyon (1990, February 25). The dream doctor Rosalind Cartwright believes dreams hold the key to curing depression. *Sun Tribune.*

S. R. Lloyd, & R. Cartwright (1995). The collection of home and laboratory dreams by means of an instrumental response technique. *Dreaming, 5*(2), 63–73.

C. A. Magee, L. D. Robinson, & A. McGregor (2018). The work-family interface and sleep quality. *Behavioral Sleep Medicine, 16*(6), 601–610. https://doi.org/10.1080/15402002.2016.1266487

R. Moss (2009). *The secret history of dreaming.* Novato, CA: New World Library.

T. D. Nelson, K. M. Kidwell, M. Hankey, J. M. Nelson, & K. P. Espy (2019). Preschool executive control and sleep problems in early adolescence. *Behavioral Sleep Medicine, 16*(5), 494–503. https://doi.org/10.1080/15402002.2016.1228650

B.-Y. Ng, & T.-L. Lee (2008). Hypnotherapy for sleep disorders. *Annals Academy of Medicine Singapore, 37*, 683–688.

H. Nichols (2018). Why does it mean when we dream? *Medical News Today*. Retrieved November 22, 2019, https://www.medicalnewstoday.com/articles/284378

M. R. Olsen, M. Schredl, & I. Carlsson (2016). People's views on dreaming: Attitudes and subjective dream theories, with regard to age, education, and sex. *Dreaming, 26*(2), 158–168. https://doi.org/10.1037/drm00002.

M. Popova (2020). The science of sleep: Dreaming, depression, and how REM sleep regulates negative emotions. *Brain Pickings*. Retrieved March 19, 2020, from https://www.brainpickings.org/2012/08/13/the-twenty-four-hour-mind-rosalind-cartwright/

S. A. Rahman, M. A. St. Hilaire, & S. W. Lockley (2017). The effects of spectral tuning of evening ambient light on melatonin suppression, alertness and sleep. *Physiology and Behavior, 177*, 221–229.

S. Sharma (2007, April 4). Parasomnias: An overview. *The Indian Journal of Medical Research, 131*(2), 333–337.

Further Resources

N. Ambardekar (2019, July 24). *Sleep disorders dictionary.* Retrieved April 21, 2021, from www.webmd.com/sleep-disorders/sleep-disorders-glossary

American Academy of Sleep Medicine. *Obstructive sleep apnea.* https://aasm.org/resources/factsheets/sleepapnea.pdf

American Chronic Pain Association. 800-533-3231. https://www.theacpa.org.

American Pain Foundation. https://www.painfoundation.org

EdenSleep. *How does CPAP work?.* https://shop.edensleep.co.nz/how-does-cpap-work/

Institute of Medicine. 2008. *Sleep disorders and sleep deprivation: An unmet public health problem.* Washington, DC: The National Academies Press. https://www.nap.edu/catalog/11617.html.

MedlinePlus. *Central sleep apnea.* MedlinePlus: National Library of Medicine (NLM). https://medlineplus.gov/ency/article/003997.htm.

National Fibromyalgia Association. https://www.fmaware.org.

National Pain Foundation. https://www.painconnection.org.

K. Sexton-Radek (2008). *Sleep quality in young adults.* New York: Mellon Publishers.

K. Sexton-Radek & G. Graci (2016). *Combating sleep disorders.* New York: Pergamon Press.

M. J. Thorpy & J. Yarger (2001). *The encyclopedia of sleep and sleep disorders* (2nd ed.). New York: Facts on File, Inc.

Index

academic stress, 123–124
active sleep, 131
alertness, 9, 37, 99, 103, 104, 115, 123, 126
allergy, 24
all-night sleep study, 46
American Academy of Pediatrics (AAP), recommended sleep for children, 109–110
apnea, 17, 23–32, 56, 83, 88, 91, 104, 113, 114, 118, 119, 134, 165
   case studies, 32–38
apnea hypopnea index, 24, 26
asthma, 24

Band-Aid approach, medication, 137
behavioral treatments, 4, 6–8, 44, 86
bipolar disorder, 98

Cartwright, Dr. Rosalind, 29, 32, 39, 150–153, 159, 160, 161
cataplexic attacks, 96, 103
   REM like activity, 96
cataplexy, 96–99, 102
chemotherapy and radiation treatment, 136

children, 5, 16–18, 104, 109, 110, 112–114, 141, 142, 152, 157
   CBT, 115
   medical management, 117
   OSA, 24
   parasomnias, 86
   pediatric sleep disorders, 113, 114
   6–12 year olds, 109
   sleep apnea, 118
   sleep hygiene, 116
   sleep problems, 115
classic migraine headache, 46
cognitive behavioral therapy, 4, 5, 44, 59, 66, 72, 85, 101, 115, 138, 141, 155
confusional arousals, 82, 83, 100

daydreaming, 89
daytime naps, 7, 99, 103, 111

Diagnostic and Statistical Manual of Mental Disorders, Fifth Edition (*DSM-5*), 2, 133
dreaming, 149–153
   case studies, 152–158

electroencephalogram (EEG), 1, 110
excessive daytime sleepiness, 17, 95, 99, 100, 114

fetus, 110

guided imagery, 8, 18, 19, 48, 66, 76, 85, 102, 134

healthy sleep habits, 99, 135
hypnosis, 8, 17, 19, 84, 85, 88
hypocretin, 46, 97
hypopnea, 22, 23, 24, 25, 26, 131, 132, 135
hypothalamic regulation
   of sleep wake state, 97

insomnia, 1–9, 26, 45, 70, 99, 113–117, 126, 132–139, 142
   case studies, 11–19
   examples, 9–10
International Classification System of Sleep Disorders (ICSD), 2
irregular sleep patterns, 123

late-night studying, 125

major depressive disorder, 98
medical costs, 72, 100
medication, 11, 17, 29, 37, 47, 50–57, 64–68, 71–75, 84–86, 99, 102–105, 117, 128, 135, 136, 137, 139, 142, 143
medication management, 67
mental health, 25, 44
movement, 4, 7, 25, 36, 37, 38, 39, 42, 66, 67, 74, 77, 86, 123, 131, 136, 137
multiple sleep latency test (MSLT), 34, 35, 37, 98, 99, 100, 104

narcolepsy, 95–100
   case studies, 100–105
night terrors, 83
nightmares, 82, 85, 112, 115, 134, 152, 153
NREM (non-rapid eye movement), 1–2, 35, 50, 81–83, 97, 110, 118, 150

observational cross-sectional study, 47
obstructive sleep apnea (OSA), 23, 56, 83, 104, 113, 114, 118–120, 134
oncology and sleep, 131–140
   case studies, 140–143
orexin, 97, 98
oximeter, 27

pacing, 67, 73
pain, 3, 8, 29, 30, 35, 36, 37, 38, 45, 47, 134, 136, 137, 142, 143
   chronic, 63–76
   complaints, 65, 70, 73, 118, 127, 132, 133, 134, 140
pain and sleep, 63–72
   case studies, 72–76
parasomnias, 81–88, 113, 114
   case studies, 88–92
pediatric sleep, 109–118
   case study, 118–120
   disorders, 113
periodic limb movement disorder (PLMD), 43, 44, 45, 47, 117
pharmacotherapy, 134–136 137
preferences for social activities, 113
psychoanalytic theory, 149
psychological factors, 133–134
public health concern, 123

REM (rapid eye movement), 1–2, 30, 35, 50, 81–82, 83, 96–97, 99, 100–102, 110, 112
REM behavior disorder, 84, 98
restless leg syndrome (RLS), 43–49, 66, 71, 91
   case studies, 49–57
   patients, 44, 45, 49

sleep hygiene, 4, 6, 9, 11, 12, 14, 16, 18, 44, 66, 73–76, 84, 87, 91, 99, 101, 104, 111,

115, 116, 117, 125, 138, 142, 154, 155
sleep paralysis, 49, 52, 54, 55, 82, 91, 95, 96, 97, 99, 104
sleep restriction, 5, 6, 7, 9, 13, 73, 87, 115, 138, 141
sleep specialist, 6, 23, 24, 28, 46, 76, 123, 126
sleep stages, 81, 97, 151
social media, 84, 113
stimulus control therapy (STC), 4, 9, 87, 115

student sleep, 123–126
   case study, 127–128

treatment planning, 69

urge to move, 43, 44, 45, 49, 51

well-being, 69, 150, 158
working, 11, 12, 14, 16, 30, 34, 37, 43, 52, 55, 56, 64, 75, 97, 98, 100, 102, 103, 104, 126, 157

About the Authors

Kathleen J. Sexton-Radek, PhD, DBSM, has been professor of psychology at Elmhurst College since 1987. She is a board member of several professional journals on sleep medicine/health psychology. Sexton-Radek's research involves investigations of sleep quality in young adults, assessment and treatment of sleep disorders, and the impact of technology on human sleep behaviors. She has published more than 100 peer-reviewed articles, book chapters, empirical reports, and editorials. She mentors students and alumni interested in sleep research and related projects.

Gina Graci, PhD, CBSM, is a licensed clinical psychologist and certified behavioral sleep medicine specialist, employed as a private practitioner specializing in sleep disorders and psychosocial oncology. She has conducted clinical trials with funding from both the private and public sectors. Graci has presented and published extensively in leading medical journals and has been interviewed frequently for stories in national and local print and broadcast media.